T0195438

INTEGRATING SYSTEMS

CLINICAL CASES
IN ANATOMY AND
PHYSIOLOGY

INTEGRATING SYSTEMS

CLINICAL CASES IN ANATOMY AND PHYSIOLOGY

ZERINA TOMKINS

PhD (Cell Biology), MNSc, Grad Cert University Teaching, BAppSc (Hons),
BAppSc (MedLabSc), MACN
Degree Coordinator (MNSc),
Department of Nursing and Department of Paediatrics,
University of Melbourne, Victoria, Australia

ELSEVIER

ELSEVIER

Elsevier Australia. ACN 001 002 357
(a division of Reed International Books Australia Pty Ltd)
Tower 1, 475 Victoria Avenue, Chatswood, NSW 2067

ISBN: 978-0-7295-4351-4

Notice

Practitioners and researchers must always rely on their own experience and knowledge in evaluating and using any information, methods, compounds or experiments described herein. Because of rapid advances in the medical sciences, in particular, independent verification of diagnoses and drug dosages should be made. To the fullest extent of the law, no responsibility is assumed by Elsevier, authors, editors or contributors for any injury and/or damage to persons or property as a matter of products liability, negligence or otherwise, or from any use or operation of any methods, products, instructions, or ideas contained in the material herein.

National Library of Australia Cataloguing-in-Publication Data

---

A catalogue record for this book is available from the National Library of Australia

---

Content Strategist: Natalie Hunt
Content Project Manager: Kritika Kaushik
Copy edited by Chris Wyard
Proofread by Tim Learner
Cover and internal design by Georgette Hall
Index by SPi Global
Typeset by GW Tech
Printed in TBD

Last digit is the print number: 9   8   7   6   5   4   3   2   1

INTRODUCTION

Undergraduate and graduate entry-to-practice healthcare students are taught anatomy and physiology with limited opportunity to apply their newly found knowledge to clinical practice or to make clinical decisions. There is also little opportunity to think how individual body systems come together to maintain system homeostasis. The aim of this resource is to highlight simple scenarios based in real-life experiences that demonstrate how knowledge of anatomy and understanding of physiology help students understand integrated responses of human structure and function that lead either to the resolution of the event or an adaptation to cope with persistence of the injurious or stressful events or stimuli.

Through doing case studies, the purpose is to build foundational skills in linking concepts taught in theoretical anatomy and physiology, to apply them to explaining sequences of events observed in real-life case presentations and to provide a scientific rationale for clinical decisions made when providing evidence-based care. Many of the presented cases will be familiar to the students as they themselves might have encountered similar presentations in their clinical practice or have personally experienced similar situations (for example, food poisoning or the common cold). By applying a problem-solving approach, the idea is to improve the student's capacity to think beyond the theory covered in the classroom, hence building confidence in their own evidence-based clinical decision-making capacity.

Each chapter starts with a brief introduction to a body system as a revision of the system's structure and main functions. Thereafter, examples of clinical cases are provided, followed by questions relevant to that case scenario. Each question is then explained by relating the answer to the anatomy and physiology underlying that response.

Evidence-based care is centred on a person-centred care model. This is the underlying reason why the case studies contain people's names. However, any similarity to someone's case is purely coincidental.

CONTENTS

ABOUT THE AUTHOR

Zerina Tomkins received her Bachelor of Medical Laboratory Science from RMIT University, Melbourne with majors in clinical biochemistry and haematology. Her honours degree, under the supervision of Prof Ian Darby, was focused on wound repair and regeneration. Zerina obtained a PhD in tissue engineering from the University of Melbourne's and St Vincent's Hospital Department of Surgery and a Master's degree in nursing, also from the University of Melbourne. Zerina completed a post-Doctoral fellowship at the Institute for Physiological Chemistry and Pathobiochemistry at the University of Münster, Germany, and was a visiting scholar at the University of California, San Francisco, and the Walter and Eliza Hall Institute of Medical Research, Australia.

Prior to her current position as the Course Coordinator at the University of Melbourne, Zerina was Head of the Vascular Anomalies Research Laboratory at Murdoch Children's Research Institute and Clinical Nurse Consultant for Vascular Anomalies at the Royal Children's Hospital.

Today, Zerina continues her association with the vascular anomalies multidisciplinary research group, leads her own interdisciplinary research group and consults on vascular biology research. Her interests are focused on four areas: (i) understanding the underlying causes of vascular anomalies and vascular cancers and how the presentation of these conditions impacts on patients and their families; (ii) long-term outcomes in this patient population, including long-term surveillance, ethical and social issues through patient-partnered research; (iii) development of vascularised tissue engineering products for transplantation; and (iv) the use of health information technology to improve the quality of healthcare delivery to disadvantaged communities. Her education interests include health informatics education for health professionals and the use of health informatics to facilitate the teaching of anatomy and physiology to healthcare students.

Zerina's publications include journal articles, reviews, letters to editors, book chapters, textbooks and abstracts totalling 65 peer-reviewed publications.

REVIEWERS

Ann Framp
PhD, MAdNursPrac, GradCertAdvNurs Auck.UT, Registered Nurse NZ
Discipline Lead, University of the Sunshine Coast, QLD

Tracy Douglas
MMedSc, GradCertULT, BSc (Hons), SFHEA
Senior Lecturer, Associate Head (Learning and Teaching)
University of Tasmania, TAS

Dr Candice Pullen
PhD, GCTE, BBiomed Sc (Hons)
Discipline Lead (Clinical Measurement)
Lecturer, Anatomy and Physiology
School of Health, Medical and Applied Sciences
CQUniversity Australia, QLD

ACKNOWLEDGMENTS

The year 2020 has brought many unexpected challenges and provided us with an opportunity to learn and grow, try and fail, and sometimes succeed, but most of all to reflect (and remember) that most important to us: our own essence of why we do what we do. The essence of my 'why' is to use my knowledge and technology to better the lives of people around me. What is most important to me are my two stout supporters: my daughter Emma and my husband Andy. My first thanks are to these two amazing persons who make my life beyond what I have hoped.

I am also grateful to Natalie Hunt, who persuaded me to share my way of writing case studies to teach nursing students how anatomy and physiology apply to nursing practice. I also thank Kritika Kaushik, who coordinated the publication of this textbook and provided support during the process of writing and editing, the Copy Editor, Chris Wyard, and the Proofreader, Tim Learner.

Finally, I would like to acknowledge the reviewers, as their suggestions and comments have improved the direction of the presented case studies.

DEDICATION

This work is dedicated to all nursing students
impacted by COVID-19:

*COVID might have stopped you from being students,
but it will not stop you from becoming great clinicians
and leaders of the future. I have faith in you.*

CASE 1
A homeless man with wounds on his feet

HISTORY

Jay is a 65-year-old man who has been homeless for the past 7 years. He presented to the emergency department after he was found by a charity worker trying to dress a large laceration on his forearm that he acquired after he fell on a rusty piece of metal. In the emergency department, the laceration was stitched with 11 sutures. During suturing, the nurse noted that Jay had worn-out tennis shoes that appeared small for his feet and with soles that were partially missing. He did not wear socks and was severely malnourished. Once Jay had removed his shoes, it was also established that he had bleeding blisters over his feet. These wounds required cleaning and dressing. His tympanic temperature was 38.2°C, his blood pressure was 135/80 and his pulse was 80 beats per minute. Following risk assessment for tetanus prophylaxis, it could not be established whether Jay had had a tetanus infection in the past.

QUESTIONS

1 What cellular responses would you expect to be activated in the wound-healing response in the arm laceration?

2. What is the purpose of cleaning the blister wounds with respect to providing an optimal healing environment for skin wound closure?

3. Why would a tetanus infection be of concern in Jay's case?

4. Discuss how intact skin acts as a barrier to tetanus infection.

5. Explain the role of the innate cellular response in managing invading microorganisms in Jay's case.

6. Discuss what may be the purpose of adaptive immune cells in managing a local infection in this case.

7. Of what significance is Jay's status of being severely malnourished with respect to providing optimal healing conditions?

ANSWERS: CASE 1
A homeless man with wounds on his feet

1. In the emergency department the laceration was closed by suturing, so that the opposing edges of the wound were now next to one another. During wound healing, the wound gap is closed via a cellular and blood vessel response to the injury, followed by an acute inflammatory response characterised by cell proliferation, cell migration, deposition of new connective tissue (composed mainly of collagen) and contraction of the newly deposited connective tissue to develop a scar. The healing process is facilitated by cells within the skin and the vascular, lymphatic, neuronal, blood (haematological), immune and endocrine systems (Figure 1.1).

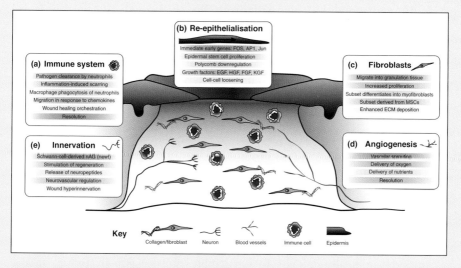

FIGURE 1.1 Cellular responses to wound healing.

The response from the skin cells includes responses in the dermal and epidermal layers. In the epidermis, skin keratinocytes at the wound edges will proliferate and migrate to seal the wound gap. In the dermis, the connective tissue cells, fibroblasts will be activated to migrate and secrete collagen to form scar tissue to close the gap.

Blood vessels have been severed in this case, due to mechanical injury, and they initially bleed into the wound gap to form a fibrin clot. Endothelial cells lining the blood vessels divide and develop a dense network of new blood vessels through a process termed angiogenesis. Similarly, the lymphatic endothelial cells lining the lymphatic vessels respond through a process of lymphangiogenesis.

The cells of the haematological system that respond to form a fibrin clot comprise erythrocytes, leukocytes, platelets and coagulation factors, the last of which are the major drivers of fibrin polymerisation. Leukocytes trapped in the fibrin clot secrete various growth factors and pro-inflammatory molecules to initiate the acute inflammatory response, including the activation of the immune system and growth of dermal connective tissue, blood vessels and neurons needed for wound repair. Mast cells play a role in regulation of the acute inflammatory response and the response of the vasculature. When the wound is formed, the mast cells secrete histamine to cause transient constriction then vasodilation of local blood vessels; this is followed by an increase in vascular permeability due to mast cell-secreted histamine and vascular endothelial growth.

Neutrophils and macrophages both phagocytose pathogens (Figure 1.2). While neutrophils kill microorganisms directly through internal processes, the macrophages process the microorganisms and present a fragment of the microorganism to the T cells in the immune organs, such as lymph nodes, to initiate adaptive immunity. Macrophages also participate in the regulation of cell processes that direct new connective tissue deposition by connective tissue fibroblasts found in the dermis, and they clean up cellular debris.

The skin is also an endocrine organ as epidermal keratinocytes produce cholecalciferol, a precursor of calcitriol, commonly known as vitamin D. This vitamin supports skin repair mechanisms.

2. Cleaning the blister wounds on the feet removes contaminants such as microorganisms and foreign materials that may be embedded in the wound bed. During wound cleaning, tissue debris and dead cells still anchored to the wound bed would be removed, hence enabling the underlying healthier cells to participate more easily in tissue repair. Failure to remove foreign bodies from the wound bed may lead to a formation of a foreign body reaction (Figure 1.2), part of a chronic acute inflammation response, which is the immune system's means of walling off a foreign body into fibrous tissue. The aim of this response is to isolate and remove non-self material. Inadequate cleaning of the wound bed will increase the risk of wound infection, which will impair wound healing.

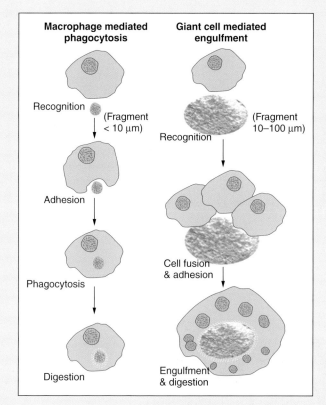

FIGURE 1.2 Foreign body reaction. For particles that are less than 10 μm in diameter, the macrophages will phagocytose the particle and process it for internal digestion. For particles that are between 10 and 100 μm in diameter, the macrophages fuse to form giant cells. The giant cells then engulf the particle and attempt to digest the material.

3. Tetanus is caused by a bacterial toxin produced by spores of the bacterium *Clostridium tetani* (Figure 1.3). As Jay's shoes are not protecting his feet, there is a possibility that the spores of this bacterium, which is found in soil, may enter the wound and develop into bacteria. The bacteria then produce a toxin called tetanospasmin, which has a neurotoxic effect (i.e. it impairs the nerves that regulate muscle contraction by blocking the release of glycine and gamma-aminobutyric acid (GABA) neurotransmitters). This is clinically evident as muscle stiffness and uncontrollable muscle spasms. Tetanus can lead to serious complications that may ultimately be fatal.

4. For *C. tetani* spores to enter the body interior, there would need to be a point of entry through the epidermis and then the dermis. However, healthy skin, which is a component of innate non-specific immunity, provides a mechanical barrier through strong keratinocyte cell-to-cell junctions that make this tissue layer impermeable to microorganisms (Figure 1.4). Keratinocytes express pattern-recognition receptors, called Toll-like receptors, which enables them to detect highly conserved

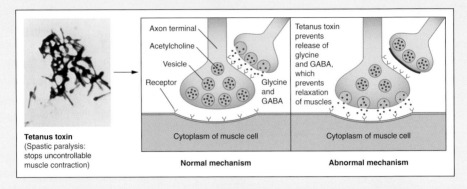

FIGURE 1.3 Mechanism of tetanus toxin in inducing uncontrollable muscle contractions.

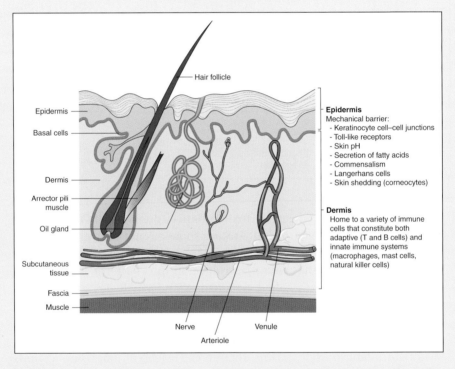

FIGURE 1.4 Skin as a primary barrier to pathogens: the epidermis and the dermis play active roles in preventing infections as well as in activating immune responses.

molecules expressed by pathogenic microorganisms. They can also secrete chemical messengers that facilitate communication with the immune system. Other skin substances include fatty acids that create a slightly acidic pH, which inhibits the growth of many pathogenic microorganisms. The skin epidermal–dermal junction area is a home to a variety of immune cells including epidermal dendritic cells (Langerhans cells), which act as antigen-presenting cells, and intraepidermal lymphocytes, which have a similar function to T cells. Keratinocytes are also shed off the skin surface and, when this occurs, microorganisms are shed at the same time. The skin is colonised by non-pathogenic bacteria, which also produce substances that inhibit the growth of many pathogenic microorganisms. In the dermis, macrophages and mast cells also aid the skin's immune function.

5. The main roles of the innate immune cellular system, in Jay's case, are to activate acute inflammation processes and to engage adaptive immune responses at the site of injury, hence effectively promoting tissue repair process while minimising the potential for infection. The innate immune cells of importance are the mast cells, macrophages, neutrophils, natural killer (NK) cells, dendritic cells, basophils and eosinophils. These cells are activated directly by the pathogen through exposure to pathogenic molecules expressed on their cell surface that are unique to those organisms. The function of each of these cells in the early innate cellular response is demonstrated in a concept map (Figure 1.5).

6. The purpose of the adaptive immune cellular response, which is carried out mainly by T and B lymphocytes, is to help destroy the pathogen and its products, and then to form a long-term memory so that immune responses can be rapidly activated if the same pathogenic organism re-invades the body. There are two broad classes of adaptive cellular responses. The first is the T-cell-mediated immune response. The second is the antibody response, which is mediated by B cells. The antibody-mediated response is also known as the humoral response.

The cell-mediated response is characterised by the activation of phagocytes (e.g. macrophages, dendritic cells), which ingest foreign bodies and then present antigens from the digested microorganism on their surface, together with MHC class II molecules. Collectively these cells are called antigen-presenting cells. Naïve T cells display antigen receptors on their surface. These receptors will engage with antigen epitopes, which are expressed by antigen-presenting cells, provided that the antigen epitope fits into the T-cell antigen receptor. Once the T cell engages with the antigen-presenting cells, it becomes activated. This leads to repeated cell mitotic division and formation of T-cell clones. It also leads to secretion of cytokines by the T-cell clones. A subset of these clones will become effector T cells. Effector T cells are cytotoxic T cells or killer T cells. Another subset of clones will form memory T cells. These memory T cells retain the information needed should the body experience another such infection. In this case, the memory T cells will differentiate into effector T cells (Figure 1.6A).

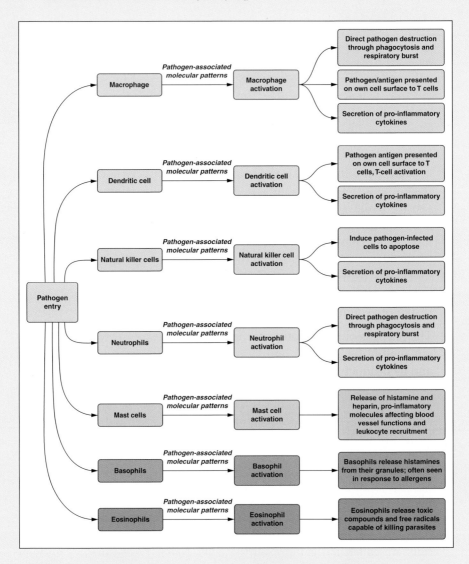

FIGURE 1.5 A concept map of innate cellular responses to pathogen entry.

The activation of B cells is initiated by the encounter between a naïve B cell (i.e. one that has never before been exposed to an antigen) and its specific antigen, (i.e. whose characteristic is that its epitope can fit the B-cell surface antibody). This initiates a series of mitotic divisions, which leads to a production of B-cell clones. Some of these clones will differentiate to become plasma B cells (effector B cells), whereas others will become memory B cells. Plasma cells will synthesise antibodies

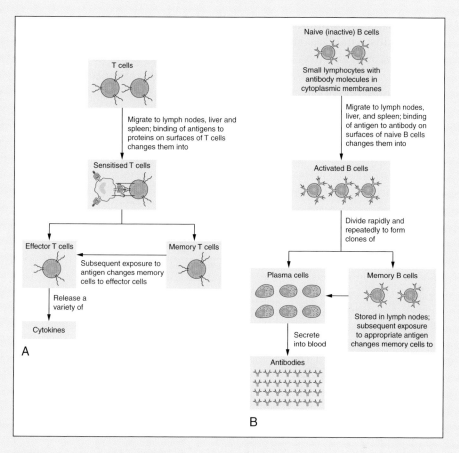

FIGURE 1.6 Adaptive immune responses. **A** General mechanisms of cell-mediated immunity. **B** A general mechanism of antibody-mediated immunity.

that will directly opsonise the antigen circulating in the blood for destruction. Memory B cells will not produce antibodies. However, if they encounter the antigen again in the future, they will rapidly divide to form new plasma cells and memory B cells to eliminate the antigen and will retain the memory of the encounter to initiate future rapid responses (Figure 1.6B).

7. Cells and their products are composed of building blocks that are derived from chemical elements, mostly derived from food intake (nutritional intake). During wound healing all cells will engage in cell proliferation, migration and specific functions (e.g. immune responses, angiogenesis, etc.). These processes require extra energy (calories) as well as building blocks to make new cells or tissue structures, or deposit extracellular

matrix. These building blocks include carbohydrates, amino acids and lipids; vitamins, such as vitamins A and C, and minerals, such as zinc, calcium and iron, are also derived from nutrition (see Figure 1.7). Malnutrition produces a systemic effect (i.e. the absence of nutrients is present in every part of the body). Protein deficiency arising from

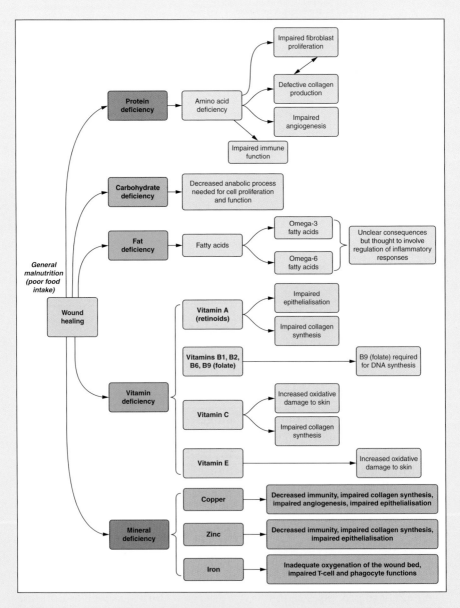

FIGURE 1.7 A concept map highlighting how nutritional deficiencies impact on wound healing.

amino acid deficiency (such as that of arginine and glutamine) is associated with delayed wound healing through delayed angiogenesis and collagen production and impacts on the immune cell function. Vitamin C is also important in collagen production and synthesis. Carbohydrates are needed to synthesise hormones and growth factors, which are important for cell proliferation, differentiation and function. This information is presented in the concept map in Figure 1.7.

BIBLIOGRAPHY

Abdelkader, A., & Barbagallo, M. S. (2020). Immune system. In Z. Tomkins (Ed.) *Applied anatomy and physiology – an interdisciplinary approach.* (1st ed.) (pp. 265–278). Chatswood, NSW: Elsevier.

Kapp, S., & Tomkins, Z. (2020). Integumentary system. In Z. Tomkins (Ed.) *Applied anatomy and physiology – an interdisciplinary approach.* (1st ed.) (pp. 53–70). Chatswood, NSW: Elsevier.

Lang, E. (2020). Nutrition and metabolism. In Z. Tomkins (Ed.) *Applied anatomy and physiology – an interdisciplinary approach.* (1st ed.) (pp. 349–360). Chatswood, NSW: Elsevier.

Quain, A. M., & Khardori, N. M. (2015). Nutrition in wound care management: a comprehensive overview. *Wounds,* 27(12), 327–335.

Rodrigues, M., Kosaric, N., Bonham, C. A., & Gurtner, G. C. (2019). Wound healing: a cellular perspective. *Physiological Reviews,* 99(1), 665–706.

The Royal Children's Hospital Melbourne. Wound assessment and management. Available at: https://www.rch.org.au/rchcpg/hospital_clinical_guideline_index/Wound_assessment_and_management/.

Tomkins, Z. (2020). Acute inflammation. In Z. Tomkins (Ed.) *Applied anatomy and physiology – an interdisciplinary approach.* (1st ed.) (pp. 279–304). Chatswood, NSW: Elsevier.

Yap, K. (2020). Nervous system. In Z. Tomkins (Ed.) *Applied anatomy and physiology – an interdisciplinary approach.* (1st ed.) (pp. 113–134). Chatswood, NSW: Elsevier.

CASE 2
A teenager with swollen lymph nodes

HISTORY

Twelve-year-old Tara and her 10-year-old sister Janet were running through fields at their grandparents' farm when Tara stepped on a piece of an old window frame lying in the tall grass. The frame had residue of glass on it and a nail embedded in it. She felt a sharp pain and, when she looked at her foot, she saw that there was a large gash in the middle of the arch of the right foot. With Janet's help, Tara returned to the farmhouse, where her grandmother helped stop the bleeding, washed the wound and bandaged it in a gauze dressing. Three days after the injury, Tara developed a fever (38.7°C) and felt generally unwell. When she went to the toilet, she noticed a painful swelling in her right groin. When she placed her hand on the swelling, she felt a strong pulse and the swelling was warm to the touch. When she showed her grandmother the swelling, the grandmother estimated it to be 1 cm in diameter. She also had a closer look at the rest of Tara's leg and noticed another mass behind the knee. This mass was also painful and warm to touch. Concerned about the discovery of these masses, the grandmother booked an appointment with the family's general practitioner (GP) and called the girls' mother.

On examination in the GP's office, Tara's tympanic temperature was 38.9°C, her blood pressure was 115/75 and her pulse was 70 beats per minute. She was shivering and she stated that she was feeling cold.

QUESTIONS

1. Tara has stepped on glass and a nail, which resulted in a cut. Which lines of immune defence have been broken, and why?

2. An open wound is a site where microorganisms can enter the human body. Discuss what role the lymphatic system has in limiting the migration of those microorganisms from the wound site throughout the rest of the body.

3. Explain why Tara felt a strong pulse in her right groin area.

4. On examination, the GP noted that Tara's inguinal and popliteal lymph nodes were very swollen. Considering the presenting history, explain why these lymph nodes were swollen.

5. Suggest why Tara has developed a temperature and was feeling cold, and explain the mechanism by which the body temperature increase would occur in this case.

6. Are Tara's blood pressure and heart rate of concern?

ANSWERS: CASE 2
A teenager with swollen lymph nodes

1. Tara's injury and presentation to her GP are consistent with all three lines of the immune defences being breached (Figure 2.1). The skin, which forms the first line of defence, was breached and it is a part of the non-specific innate defence system. The skin is a mechanical barrier, and skin cells secrete substances such as lysozymes, enzymes that can break down the cell wall of some bacteria, meaning that the skin is also a chemical barrier. Damage to skin epidermal and dermal layers diminish the skin's capacity to maintain these functions. The underlying connective tissue, blood vessels and lymphatic vessels would also be damaged and secrete chemical substances that activate non-specific immune responses to deal with antigen exposure – the second line of defence. This includes a cellular response by resident inflammatory cells such as macrophages and neutrophils and activation of the acute inflammatory response by the injured tissue, which helps limit tissue damage and enable tissue repair. The third line of defence is that of the adaptive immune system, which would be activated either through

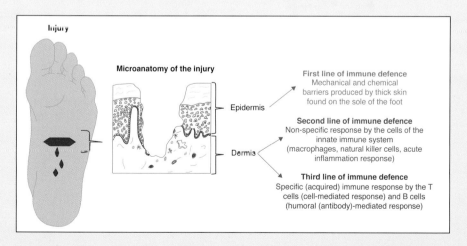

FIGURE 2.1 The formation of the wound on the foot breaches three lines of immune defence.

antigen-cell presentation to T cells (cell mediated-immunity) to activate the immune responses or through B-cell response mediated by antibody secretion specific to the microbial antigen (humoral immunity). Note that T cells can also activate B cells to produce antibodies. The evidence that the third line of defence has been activated is presented through swollen lymph nodes.

2. Microorganisms enter lymph vessels through lymphatic endothelial cell gaps of the initial lymphatic capillary and travel to a nearby lymph node as lymph is propelled unidirectionally from the site of injury from one lymph node to another (Figure 2.2). Once in the lymph node, the microorganisms would encounter the cells of the immune system, where the immune response is mounted. Microorganisms are captured at the site of entry by antigen-presenting cells (such as dendritic cells and macrophages) and carried to lymph nodes, where they are presented to local T cells for T-cell-mediated responses.

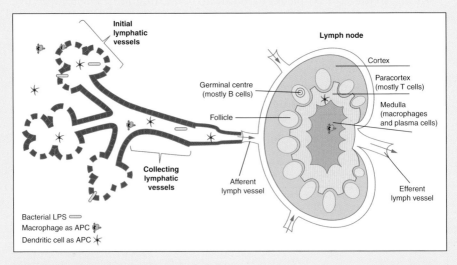

FIGURE 2.2 Mode and transport of microorganisms and antigens from the tissue periphery via initial and collecting lymphatic vessels to the local lymph node for presentation to immune cells and activation of the adaptive immune response.

3. The area where Tara has felt a swollen lymph node and strong pulse is an area where the femoral artery is found (Figure 2.3). This is a large artery that supplies arterial (oxygenated) blood to the thigh and leg (the lower extremities).

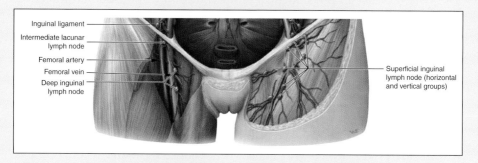

FIGURE 2.3 The anatomical relationship between the femoral artery and the inguinal lymph nodes.

4. The observation at the time of the clinical assessment that the popliteal and inguinal lymph nodes were swollen suggests that the immune response has been activated (Figure 2.4). As lymph nodes are home to both T and B cells, it is expected that each would engage with the presenting antigens/microorganisms via mechanisms unique to those cells. For example, microorganisms that were captured and taken to lymph nodes by antigen-presenting cells are presented to T cells, which recognise the foreign antigen on the surface of the antigen-presenting cell. T cells respond by undergoing a process of clonal division, dividing into many T cells with identical capability of tackling that specific antigen. B cells will engage

FIGURE 2.4 Swelling of a lymph node following clonal expansion of T and B cells.

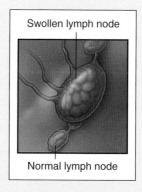

directly with the microorganisms and undergo a clonal division process. The consequence of this cell division is that the lymph node grows to accommodate new T and B cells. Thus, on palpation, these lymph nodes would be larger.

5. The increase in physiological temperature in response to an infection involves the immune system, peripheral and central nervous system, vascular system, muscular system, cutaneous system and endocrine system (Figure 2.5). Upon exposure to pathogen-derived molecules – for example, microbial products such as lipopolysaccharides (structural elements of the bacterial cell wall) – or viruses, the innate immune cells (such as macrophages and dendritic cells) will release prostaglandin E2 (PGE2), a major pyrogenic mediator of fever, and pyrogenic cytokines such as interleukin-1 (IL-1), interleukin-6 (IL-6) and tumour necrosis factor (TNF), which will collectively induce systemic fever. PGE2 is produced at the site of infection by the injured tissue and by the brain's vascular endothelial cells and it travels via the blood–brain barrier to bind to prostaglandin receptors expressed by thermoregulatory neurons within the hypothalamus. There, the core temperature of the body will be reset to a higher level. The neurotransmitter noradrenaline (norepinephrine) is released, which causes vasoconstriction via arteriolar smooth muscle cells that prevents heat loss. Noradrenaline will also be released by the adrenaline gland. The neurotransmitter acetylcholine is also released to stimulate skeletal muscles to produce heat through an increased metabolic rate, which is visible to us as shivering. Thyroxine is released by the thyroid gland to help increase the metabolic rate to meet the increased metabolic demand needed to maintain the physiological processes during fever. If the temperature reaches too high a point, the hypothalamus will also direct sweat glands in the skin to release sweat and cause relaxation of the erector pili muscle, which should cause increased heat evaporation. This leads to a behavioural change – for example, asking for a blanket to keep warm. IL-1, IL-6 and TNF are also thought to influence the hypothalamus. The hypothalamus receives input from receptors in the skin (cutaneous nerves) that control external temperature and receptors in the hypothalamus (which control and oversee the body's core temperature). The benefit of the fever is to enhance immune mechanisms combating the infection through promoting innate and adaptive immune responses.

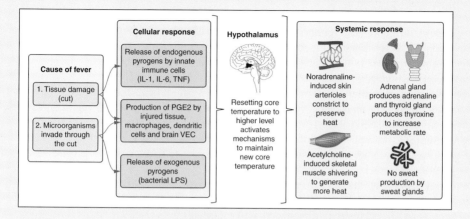

FIGURE 2.5 Initial response by the hypothalamus in increasing core body temperature in response to microorganism invasion and mechanical tissue injury. IL-1 = interleukin-1, IL-6 = interleukin-6, LPS = lipopolysaccharide, TNF = tumour necrosis factor, VEC = vascular endothelial cells.

6. Tara's blood pressure and pulse should be considered with caution for two reasons:

   a. there is no baseline measure to let us know what the blood pressure and pulse was prior to her becoming unwell, so there is nothing to compare it with;

   b. the values are within the normal reference range and as such may not be viewed as a concern.

Caution: it is important not to take reference values blindly. Instead, they need to be applied in a person-centred manner. For example, if a person's usual blood pressure is 90/55 mmHg then pressure of 125/80 may be of significance. This baseline can sometimes be established if the clinician asks the patient whether they know their usual blood pressure.

BIBLIOGRAPHY

Abdelkader, A., & Barbagallo, M. S. (2020). Immune system. In Z. Tomkins (Ed.) *Applied anatomy and physiology – an interdisciplinary approach.* (1st ed.) (pp. 265–278). Chatswood, NSW: Elsevier.

Evans, S. S., Repasky, E. A., & Fisher, D. T. (2015). Fever and the thermal regulation of immunity: the immune system feels the heat. *Nature Reviews. Immunology,* 15(6), 335–349. doi: 10.1038/nri3843.

Jackson, D. (2019). Leukocyte trafficking via the lymphatic vasculature – mechanisms and consequences. *Frontiers in Immunology*, 10, 471. doi: 10.3389/fimmu.2019.00471.

Kapp, S., & Tomkins, Z. (2020). Integumentary system. In Z. Tomkins (Ed.) *Applied anatomy and physiology – an interdisciplinary approach.* (1st ed.) (pp. 53–70). Chatswood, NSW: Elsevier.

Nelson, S., & Tomkins, Z. (2020). Cardiovascular system. In Z. Tomkins (Ed.) *Applied anatomy and physiology – an interdisciplinary approach.* (1st ed.) (pp. 227–248). Chatswood, NSW: Elsevier.

Tomkins, Z. (2020). Acute inflammation. In Z. Tomkins (Ed.) *Applied anatomy and physiology – an interdisciplinary approach.* (1st ed.) (pp. 279–304). Chatswood, NSW: Elsevier.

Tomkins, Z., & Phillips, J. (2020). Lymphatic system and tissue fluid balance maintenance. In Z. Tomkins (Ed.) *Applied anatomy and physiology – an interdisciplinary approach.* (1st ed.) (pp. 249–264). Chatswood, NSW: Elsevier.

CASE 3
A motor scooter rider with multiple closed fractures of the femur

HISTORY

Jamie was riding a 200-watt motor scooter at 10 kilometres per hour when she was hit by a small SUV travelling at 40 kilometres an hour. She was lifted off of her scooter and was thrown into the air onto concrete. At the time of the accident, Jamie wore a helmet and knee and elbow pads. A quick-thinking bystander called for an ambulance while another rushed to secure the scene and provide first aid. Jamie did not lose consciousness, but was in a lot of pain screaming that she might have broken her left leg. On assessment, the paramedic suspected that Jamie had multiple fractures in her left leg as the paramedic also observed an anterior swelling approximately 5 centimetres below the patella. There were no bones protruding through the skin; however, the paramedic could not be sure whether some of the fractures might be displaced. To alleviate Jamie's pain and help prepare her for the transport to the hospital, one of the paramedics inserted an intravenous needle and administered painkillers intravenously. Once the painkillers were effective, Jamie's leg was immobilized; then she was moved onto a stretcher, into the ambulance and taken to the hospital.

QUESTIONS

1. Why is it significant that the fractured femur is a closed fracture and not an open fracture?

2. As the femur has not broken through the skin, discuss what other damage to the surrounding tissue is expected in this case.

3. Considering that, on assessment, the paramedic also observed a swelling approximately 5 centimetres below the patella, which other bones might be fractured in Jamie's case?

4. Explain the haematological response when a bone is fractured.

5. Discuss how the femur will repair over the next 6 to 8 weeks and why it was important to immobilise the femur at the time of fracture.

6. The leg is immobilised with a cast to allow the bone to repair. If the cast had been made incorrectly, what might occur to the encased limb?

ANSWERS: CASE 3
A motor scooter rider with multiple closed fractures of the femur

1. Closed fractures will need to be treated differently from open fractures (Figure 3.1). This is because the overlying skin is not broken; therefore, the first line of defence is not broken. Hence, dirt and bacteria in the environment cannot enter the area of the wound, so infection is not likely to occur owing to the accident.

2. This bone fracture may involve damage to surrounding muscle, blood and lymphatic vascular systems as well as to local nerves. One possible form of damage is mechanical severing of these structures. The other is compression injury. The significance of this being a closed fracture is that the blood from injured bone would flow into the surrounding tissue, leading to swelling in the injured area. Acute inflammation and damage to blood vessels in the area may further damage the tissue and

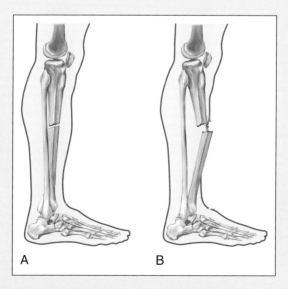

FIGURE 3.1 A Closed fracture and **B** open fracture. Note that the open fracture has bone in direct contact with the external environment.

lead to hypoxia and tissue acidosis, which may compromise the healing process. In severe cases, and if not monitored correctly, this may lead to the compartment syndrome, whereby the affected tissue cannot cope with the localised tissue swelling and the tissue starts to undergo necrosis.

3. As the swelling is anterior, this is most likely indicative that the tibia has been fractured. However, X-rays would be needed to confirm this and to exclude fracture to the fibula.

4. Long bones have their own vascular supply comprising a nutrient artery, which nourishes the diaphysis and metaphysis, the medullary cavity and the bone cortex, and periosteal and epiphyseal blood vessels. Blood is drained from the long bones by a system of veins that leave the periosteum through muscle insertions. Bone marrow (housed in the bone medulla) is highly vascularised. Following bone fracture, blood will flow into the injured area. This flow will cease shortly as, at the same time, the blood coagulation system will become activated through a process of haemostasis (which involves a complement cascade, a clotting factor cascade, platelet aggregation and vascular endothelial cell responses) and a fibrin clot will form to stop further bleeding. The clotted blood formed around the fractured bone is called a haematoma. A haematoma in the bone also acts as a provisional matrix for inflammatory cells (macrophages, polymorphonuclear cells) and local tissue cells (fibroblasts) to respond to the injury and commence repair in the first few days of injury (Figure 3.2).

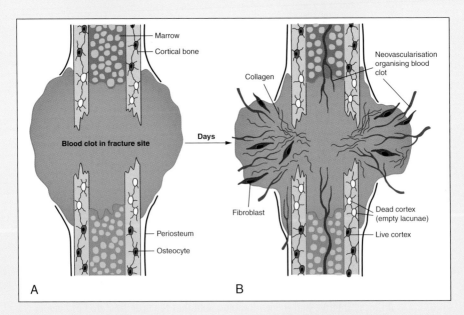

FIGURE 3.2 A A blood clot acts as a provisional matrix **B** for tissue cells to initiate bone repair.

5. Bone fracture leads to bleeding arising from damage to periosteal blood
    vessels. Blood pools at the site of injury, and the clotting system activates
    the formation of the fibrin matrix, which will provide a scaffold for local
    cells to migrate, differentiate and form new bone (Figure 3.3A, B). Initially,
    these cells give rise to a cartilaginous tissue mass, the procallus, whose role
    is to act as a glue that anchors the two opposing bone ends (Figure 3.3C). In
    time, the procallus is replaced by bony callus tissue, which binds the broken

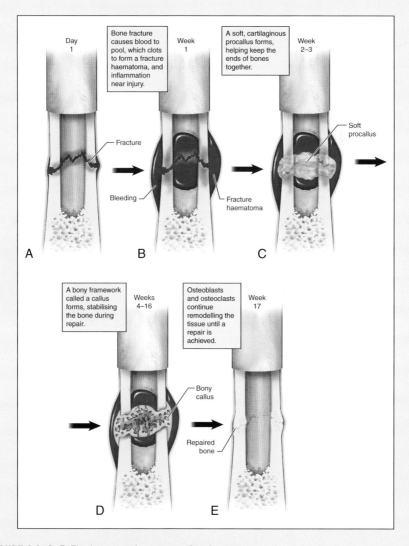

FIGURE 3.3 A–E. The bone repair process after fracture.
A–C: Courtesy of Dennis Strete; **D, E:** From Kumar, V., & Abbas, A. (2005). *Robbins and Cotran pathologic basis of disease*. Philadelphia, PA: Saunders.

ends more securely while allowing the formation of the bone marrow cavity (Figure 3.3D). During this process, the bone is fragile and cannot take weight-bearing activities, so immobilising the bone protects the newly formed bone. Eventually, bony callus is replaced by the repaired calcified bone (Figure 3.3E). By immobilising the leg, the bone is given time to repair. If the bone is not immobilised, it may lead to deformity of the healed bone, which would affect weight-bearing capacity, mobility and gait.

6. Part of the acute inflammatory response and the bone repair process is swelling. If the cast is applied too tightly, then the tissue will have a very limited space to increase in size as it swells. This means that the swelling may compress local tissue, blood vessels and nerves, leading to loss of oxygen perfusion, loss of innervation and increase in tissue hypoxia and acidosis. If unrelieved, this can lead to tissue death and loss of the limb. This condition is known as compartment syndrome (Figure 3.4) and it is a medical emergency.

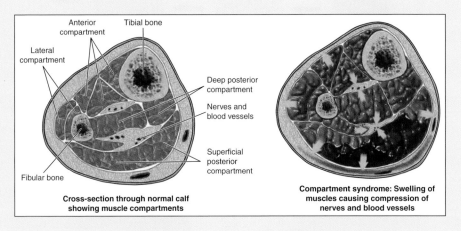

FIGURE 3.4 Compartment syndrome.

BIBLIOGRAPHY

Abdelkader, A., & Barbagallo, M. S. (2020). Immune system. In Z. Tomkins (Ed.) *Applied anatomy and physiology – an interdisciplinary approach.* (1st ed.) (pp. 265–278). Chatswood, NSW: Elsevier.

Lee, M. (2020). Muscular system. In Z. Tomkins (Ed.) *Applied anatomy and physiology – an interdisciplinary approach.* (1st ed.) (pp. 103–112). Chatswood, NSW: Elsevier.

Loi, F., Córdova, L. A., Pajarinen, J., Lin, T. H., Yao, Z., & Goodman, S. B. (2016). Inflammation, fracture and bone repair. Bone, 86, 119–130. doi: 10.1016/j.bone. 2016.02.020.

Moore, S. (2020). The skeletal system. In Z. Tomkins (Ed.) *Applied anatomy and physiology – an interdisciplinary approach.* (1st ed.) (pp. 71–86). Chatswood, NSW: Elsevier.

Newall, F., & Tomkins, Z. (2020). Haemostasis. In Z. Tomkins (Ed.) *Applied anatomy and physiology – an interdisciplinary approach.* (1st ed.) (pp. 209–226). Chatswood, NSW: Elsevier.

Tomkins, Z. (2020). Acute inflammation. In Z. Tomkins (Ed.) *Applied anatomy and physiology – an interdisciplinary approach.* (1st ed.) (pp. 279–304). Chatswood, NSW: Elsevier.

Tomlinson, R. E., & Silva, M. J. (2013). Skeletal blood flow in bone repair and maintenance. *Bone Research,* 1(4), 311–322. doi: 10.4248/BR201304002.

Tull, F., & Borrelli, J., Jr (2003). Soft-tissue injury associated with closed fractures: evaluation and management. *Journal of American Academy of Orthopedic Surgeons,* 11(6), 431–438.

CASE 4

An infant with overgrowth of the right brain hemisphere

HISTORY

A 3-month-old girl, Sarah, was diagnosed with an overgrowth of her right brain hemisphere (right hemimegaloencephaly). Sarah was born full term with no birth-related complications. However, within 2 months of birth she started to suffer from seizures. She was referred to the children's hospital neurologists for further investigations. The seizures increased in intensity and frequency as she grew older and could not be controlled by medications. The positron emission tomography (PET) scan showed that she had two abnormal spots on her right hemisphere. One spot was on the parietal lobe and the other overlapped a portion of the primary motor cortex. To ease the seizures, surgeons decided to remove 80% of the right cerebral cortex, sparing areas crucial to vision, hearing and sensory processing. They also removed the motor cortex. A sample of the removed tissue was sent to the pathology lab for genetic testing. This test revealed that the affected brain tissue contained a somatic mosaic mutation in the gene *PIK3CA*, which leads to tissue overgrowth.

QUESTIONS

1. In which lobe are the centres for vision, hearing and sensory processing respectively?

2. Which abilities would you expect Sarah to lose with the removal of the right hemisphere?

3. Which abilities would be impaired if the left hemisphere were taken out instead?

4. If only the cortex of the right hemisphere was removed, which parts of the cerebrum did the surgeons leave behind?

5. Why did the surgeons spare Sarah's right lateral ventricle?

6. Explain the importance of the diagnosis being that of a somatic mutation rather than a germline mutation.

ANSWERS: CASE 4
An infant with overgrowth of the right brain hemisphere

1. The centre for vision is located in the occipital lobe (Figure 4.1). The centre for hearing is located in the temporal lobe and the centre for processing of sensory information (e.g. temperature, taste, touch, movement) is predominantly located in the parietal lobe.

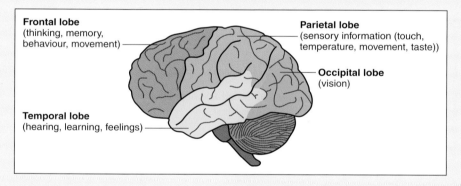

FIGURE 4.1 Lobes of the brain.

2. The right brain hemisphere is responsible for coordination of left-sensory and motor functions (Figure 4.2), so Sarah would be expected to experience impairment of those functions.

3. Removal of the left hemisphere would impair Sarah's speech ability, as Wernicke's area and Broca's area are both located in the left hemisphere (see Figure 4.2). Right ear hearing would be affected, as the auditory cortex for the right ear would be removed. The general interpretative centre for language and mathematics would also be impacted.

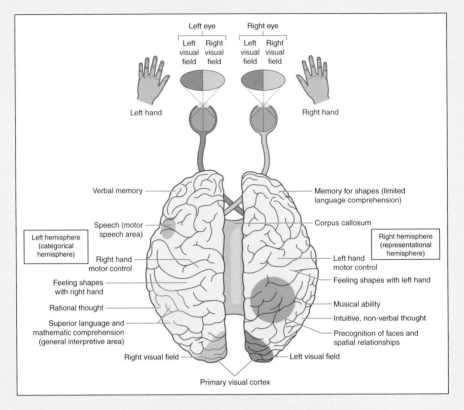

FIGURE 4.2 Functional specialisations of the left and right brain hemispheres.
Copyright ©McGraw-Hill Companies Inc., with permission.

4. The surgeons would leave behind the white matter, interior nuclei and ventricles (see Figure 4.3).

5. The walls of ventricles (Figure 4.3) contain the choroid plexus, which secretes cerebrospinal fluid (CSF). CSF plays a protective role by cushioning the brain. Without CSF, there would be a potential for brain damage from jarring of the head. CSF also plays a role in acid–base balance.

6. A somatic mutation occurs after a zygote is formed and it is not inherited from either parent. Somatic mutations cannot be passed to one's offspring, which is characteristic for germline mutations (Figure 4.4). Another characteristic of the somatic mutation is that only the cells that arose from the mutated cell will contain that mutation, whereas the rest of the cells will be mutation free. The earlier the somatic mutation occurs during embryonic development, the greater its distribution. In contrast, germline mutations are present in all body and germ cells.

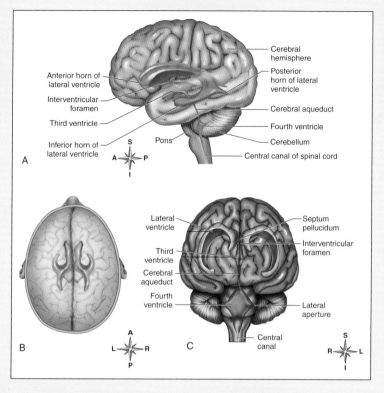

FIGURE 4.3 A Left lateral view of the brain ventricles (highlighted in blue). **B** View of the brain ventricles from above. **C** View of the brain ventricles from the front.

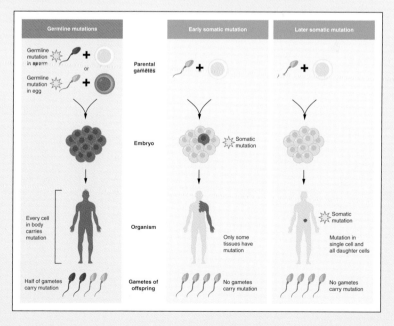

FIGURE 4.4 Comparison of germline and somatic mutations.

BIBLIOGRAPHY

Lee, J. H., Huynh, M., Silhavy, J. L., Kim, S., Dixon-Salazar, T., Heiberg, A., et al. (2012). De novo somatic mutations in components of the PI3K-AKT3-mTOR pathway cause hemimegalencephaly. *Nature Genetics*, 44(8), 941–945. doi: 10.1038/ng.2329.

Madsen, R. R., Vanhaesebroeck, B., & Semple, R. K. (2018). Cancer-associated *PIK3CA* mutations in overgrowth disorders. *Trends in Molecular Medicine*, 24(10), 857–870.

Nayagam, B., & Nayagam, D. X. (2020). Special senses: hearing, balance and vision. In Z. Tomkins (Ed.) *Applied anatomy and physiology – an interdisciplinary approach.* (1st ed.) (pp. 151–168). Chatswood, NSW: Elsevier.

Tomkins, Z. (2020). Genes and genomics. In Z. Tomkins (Ed.) *Applied anatomy and physiology – an interdisciplinary approach.* (1st ed.) (pp. 29–52). Chatswood, NSW: Elsevier.

Yap, K. (2020). Nervous system. In Z. Tomkins (Ed.) *Applied anatomy and physiology – an interdisciplinary approach.* (1st ed.) (pp. 113–134). Chatswood, NSW: Elsevier.

CASE 5
Watery eye and common cold

HISTORY

Mannika is a third-year university student. This morning she woke up with a sore throat, blocked nose, watery eyes and mild sinus pain. She checked her temperature, which was 37.8°C. Mannika was concerned how her illness would impact on her studies so she visited her local clinic, where she was told that she has a common cold, a condition caused by a virus.

QUESTIONS

1. Why did Mannika experience watery eyes with a common cold?

2. What is the significance of the sinus pain?

3. Why is her nose blocked and how would this impact on her capacity to breathe?

ANSWERS: CASE 5
Watery eye and common cold

1. Normally, the lacrimal glands, which are exocrine glands located in the upper lateral region of each eye orbit, produce a fluid (commonly known as tears) that acts as a lubricant and has a role in protecting, moistening and cleaning the eye. The fluid is secreted via secretory ducts on the conjunctiva of the eye at the upper outer corner of the eye (Figure 5.1). Secreted tears gather in the fornix conjunctiva of the upper eyelid. From there the fluid is carried across the eye surface to

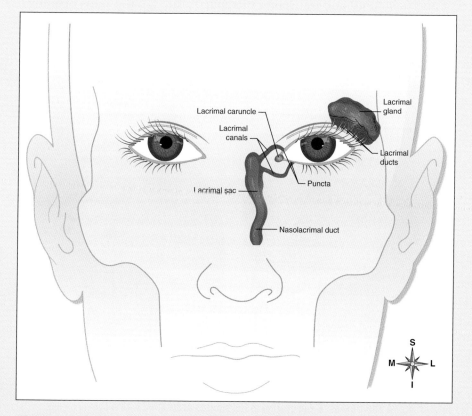

FIGURE 5.1 Formation of tears by the lacrimal gland and their conduction to the nasal cavity.

the lacrimal puncta, which are openings into the lacrimal canals and are found at the inner corner of eyelids. The lacrimal puncta duct carries tears to the lacrimal canals, lacrimal sac and nasolacrimal duct, which drains the tears into nasal cavity.

During a common cold, the virus that infects the nasal mucosal lining of the nose infects the mucosal lining of the tear ducts, as these are an extension of the nasal mucosa. This leads to localised acute inflammation characterised by oedema and swelling of the mucosa. Subsequently, the nasolacrimal ducts narrow in diameter and the flow of tear secretions is blocked. The fluid accumulates in the eye and is evident as a 'watery eye'.

2. Sinus pain during a common cold signifies that the virus has spread to the sinus membrane and caused inflammation. Sinuses are air-filled spaced cavities within a bone and are lined with mucous membranes (Figure 5.2A). Sinusoidal mucous membranes are lined with ciliated epithelium, which produces thin mucus that traps microorganisms and pollutants, and transports this mucus through the sinus openings into the nasal cavity. During infection, the epithelial-lined mucosa is inflamed, and it produces an increased volume of very thick mucus

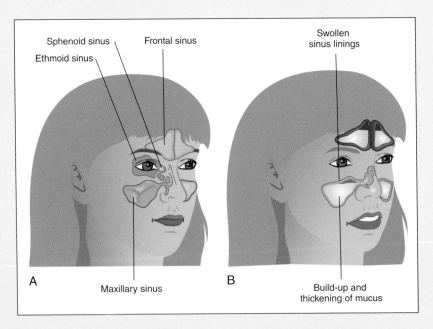

FIGURE 5.2 A The sinuses. **B** Congestion of the sinuses associated with a common cold.

(Figure 5.2B). This can lead to blockage of the sinus openings, which in turn leads to a build-up of pressure in the sinus cavities. This in turn stimulates pain receptors. The distribution of the pain depends on which sinus is affected. For example, forehead and cheek pain would be indicative of inflammation of the frontal and maxillary sinuses respectively.

3. During common cold, the ciliated epithelium of the nasal cavity would produce thick mucus that has trapped infectious viral particles. Furthermore, sinus drainage would empty the mucus into the nasal cavity. This thick mucus builds up and congests the nasal passage. Air passage through the congested pathway is obstructed and the person may find themself breathing through the mouth.

BIBLIOGRAPHY

Battisti, A. S., Modi, P., & Pangia, J. (2020). Sinusitis. In *StatPearls* [Internet]. Treasure Island, FL: StatPearls Publishing. Available from: https://www.ncbi.nlm.nih.gov/books/NBK470383/.

DeBoer D. L., & Kwon, E. (2020). Acute sinusitis. In *StatPearls* [Internet]. Treasure Island, FL: StatPearls Publishing. Available from: https://www.ncbi.nlm.nih.gov/books/NBK547701/.

Nayagam, B., & Nayagam, D. X. (2020). Special senses: hearing, balance and vision. In Z. Tomkins (Ed.) *Applied anatomy and physiology – an interdisciplinary approach.* (1st ed.) (pp. 151–168). Chatswood, NSW: Elsevier.

Tomkins, Z. (2020). Acute inflammation. In Z. Tomkins (Ed.) *Applied anatomy and physiology – an interdisciplinary approach.* (1st ed.) (pp. 279–304). Chatswood, NSW: Elsevier.

CASE 6
Formalin-loaded taste buds

HISTORY

Kiki's class went to the anatomy museum, where they saw cadavers for the entire day. Their lecturer carefully explained the anatomical function of each body part on display. Kiki thought that the class was very interesting even though she found it initially hard to stay in the museum, as the smell of formalin was overwhelming. Formalin is a compound used to preserve tissues. However, she did get used to it and by the time the morning tea break came around the smell no longer bothered her. What did bother her, however, was that, when she went to have her lunch, her sandwich and orange juice both tasted like the smell of formalin. This made her lose her appetite. She returned to the museum for an afternoon session. In the evening, she took a bus home and thought that she must smell of formalin, as that was all she could smell. She started to worry about the bus passengers, who most probably would be able to smell it too. When she got home, she was starving. Her mother made a roast beef and vegetable meal, but one taste of that and she felt again as though she were eating formalin. She stopped eating her dinner and went outside to get some fresh air. Kiki hoped that the feeling would not last for long

QUESTIONS

1. Explain why the smell of formalin initially bothered Kiki and why she got used to it.

2. Propose why everything Kiki ate tasted like formalin.

3. Which cranial nerves are involved in mediating the senses of smell and taste?

ANSWERS: CASE 6
Formalin-loaded taste buds

1. The olfactory nerve, which initially detects the formalin (stimulus, odorant) via the sensory cells, becomes desensitised with continuous exposure to formalin particles. Initially, formalin molecules would stimulate the sensory nerve and initiate the firing of impulses, which would then be conducted to the olfactory sensing region in the brain (Figure 6.1). There, the impulse would be processed and interpreted so

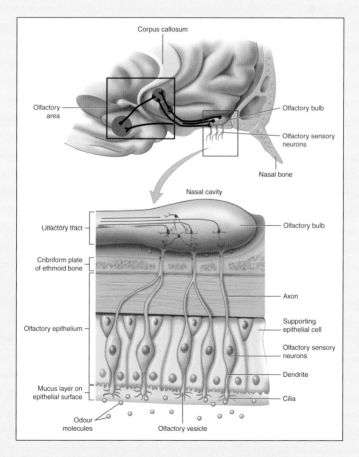

FIGURE 6.1 Detection of odour molecules by the receptors in the olfactory bulb and transmission of neuronal impulses to the brain.

that the brain could correctly interpret the stimulant and make Kiki respond appropriately. Considering that Kiki spent an entire day in the anatomy museum, where formalin was constantly present in the museum, her olfactory receptors would eventually become saturated and her brain would perceive this as a decrease in the intensity of the formalin smell and therefore it posed no danger, giving the impression that the smell is not as offensive as when first encountered.

2. Some of the formalin particles would diffuse into the mouth cavity, where they would interact with the taste buds. The taste buds are the sense organs that respond to gustatory stimuli (taste stimuli). Most taste buds are tongue papillae (Figure 6.2A). The chemoreceptors needed to interpret gustatory stimuli are located in the taste buds. They are stimulated by chemicals that are present in the mouth environment, called tastants, dissolved in the saliva. Each taste bud is like a banana-like cluster that contains 50 to 125 of these chemoreceptors (Figure 6.2B), called gustatory cells (Figure 6.2C). These cells are surrounded by a supportive epithelial cell capsule. Cilia, or gustatory hairs, project from each of the gustatory cells and extend into an opening called the taste pore, which also contains saliva. As these chemoreceptors have already been stimulated by formalin molecules, regardless of what Kiki ate her food would taste of formalin.

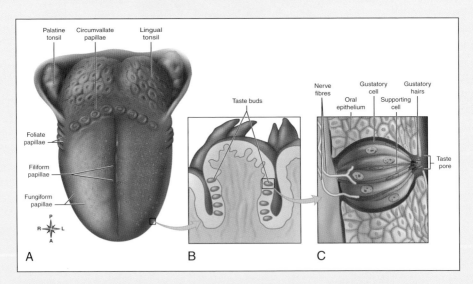

FIGURE 6.2 The tongue structure. **A** Dorsal surface of the tongue and adjacent tonsils. **B** Section through tongue papillae and side view of taste buds. **C** Section through a taste bud with supporting cells.

3. The taste sensation begins with creation of a receptor potential in the gustatory cells of a taste bud. The generation and propagation of an action potential, or nerve impulse, then transmits the sensory input to the brain. Nerve impulses generated in the anterior two-thirds of the tongue travel along the facial nerve (cranial nerve (CN) VII), whereas those generated from the posterior one-third are conducted by the glossopharyngeal nerve (CN IX) (Figure 6.3). A third cranial nerve, the vagus nerve (CN X), has a minor role in the identification of taste. It contains a few fibres that carry taste sensation from a limited number of taste buds located in the walls of the pharynx and on the epiglottis. All three cranial nerves carry neuronal stimuli into the medulla oblongata. Flavour, as the term is normally used, is a combined sense of smell, taste and the so-called trigeminal senses (mediated by CN V) that detect irritants, textures and other characteristics present in spices and most other foods.

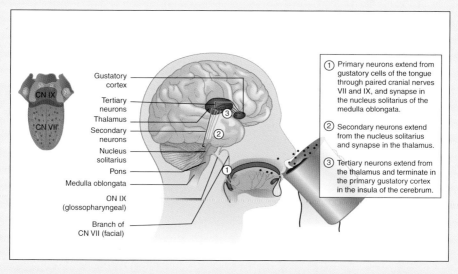

FIGURE 6.3 The gustatory pathway: (1) the facial nerve (CN VII) transmits taste sensation from the anterior two-thirds of the tongue; the glossopharyngeal nerve (CN X) transmits taste signals from the posterior one-third of the tongue. (2) These signals are transmitted to the medulla oblongata, to the region known as the nucleus solitarius, and (3) are then sent via the thalamus to the gustatory cortex in the cerebrum.

BIBLIOGRAPHY

Nayagam, B., & Nayagam, D. X. (2020). Special senses: hearing, balance and vision. In Z. Tomkins (Ed.) *Applied anatomy and physiology – an interdisciplinary approach.* (1st ed.) (pp. 151–168). Chatswood, NSW: Elsevier.

Purves, D., Augustine, G. J., Fitzpatrick, D., Katz, L. C., Lamantia, A.-S., McNamara, J. O., et al. (Eds.) (2001). *Neuroscience* (2nd ed.). (Chapter: The organization of the taste system.) Sunderland, MA: Sinauer Associates. Available from: https://www.ncbi.nlm.nih.gov/books/NBK11018/?otool=iaumelblib.

Yap, K. (2020). Nervous system. In Z. Tomkins (Ed.) *Applied anatomy and physiology – an interdisciplinary approach.* (1st ed.) (pp. 113–134). Chatswood, NSW: Elsevier.

Yap, K. (2020). Gastrointestinal system. In Z. Tomkins (Ed.) *Applied anatomy and physiology – an interdisciplinary approach.* (1st ed.) (pp. 329–348). Chatswood, NSW: Elsevier.

CASE 7
A young woman with low blood cholesterol levels

HISTORY

Geraldine is aware that her family has a strong history of heart disease and that the best way to avoid developing heart disease is to take preventative action and avoid unhealthy foods. She has stopped eating meat and avoids any foods that may contain cholesterol. Having recently applied for a new position as a registered nurse in a large tertiary hospital, Geraldine visited her GP to review her immune status. At that time, she asked her GP to do a cholesterol profile test. While she expected her cholesterol to be within the normal range, she was surprised when her GP stated that her fasting cholesterol was too low (1.0 mmol/L; reference range: 2.0–4.0 mmol/L). The GP informed Geraldine that it might be worthwhile reviewing her strict diet, as healthy cholesterol concentrations are important in human health.

QUESTIONS

1. Considering your knowledge of hormone production, cellular structure and digestive processes, suggest why cholesterol may be important in human health.

2. Discuss the dietary and non-dietary sources of cholesterol in the human body.

3. If Geraldine does not correct her cholesterol level, what consequences may eventuate? Provide a rationale for your answer.

ANSWERS: CASE 7
A young woman with low blood cholesterol levels

1. Cholesterol is important to human health as it is a building block of the cell membrane – a structure that protects the cell from its surrounding environment through its specialised structure and highly selective permeability to organic molecules and ions (Figure 7.1). Cell membranes also regulate the movement of substances from the cell interior to the environment, and vice versa. Cholesterol is a precursor molecule (substrate) needed for the synthesis of steroid hormones. For example, the sex hormones oestrogen and testosterone are important in reproduction. Glucocorticoids, cortisol and corticosterone play a role in regulating inflammation processes, while mineralocorticoids impact on

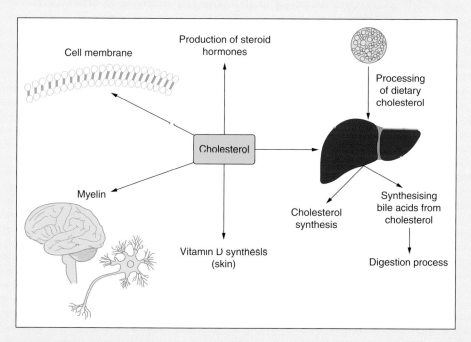

FIGURE 7.1 Uses of cholesterol in the human body.

cellular ion balance. Cholesterol is important in the production of bile acids by the liver and is needed for the digestion of fats in food. It is also a precursor molecule needed for the synthesis of vitamin D in the skin. Finally, cholesterol is important in neuronal impulse transmission as it is a building block of myelin.

2. Cholesterol is derived from both dietary and non-dietary sources. Approximately 15% is thought to be derived from dietary sources that are animal products such as dairy, eggs, meat and organs (liver and kidneys). No cholesterol is found in plant-based foods. The term 'non-dietary source of cholesterol' refers to the biosynthesis of cholesterol by the liver. This organ synthesises the remaining 85% of the body's cholesterol and is responsible for maintaining relatively constant levels of cholesterol in the blood. It synthesises cholesterol through a number of different biochemical pathways; however, one of the best understood is that of lipogenesis, in which acetyl coenzyme A (which is generated in mitochondria) is converted through a series of biochemical reactions into cholesterol.

3. Insufficient cholesterol levels may lead to impaired synthesis of all steroid hormones, which would translate to deficiencies of these hormones and abnormalities in the functions that these hormones create. Hence, reduction of or defective sex hormone synthesis could impact Geraldine's fertility. If she were to fall severely ill, her capacity to respond to critical illness may be impaired. She could also be at higher risk of intracerebral haemorrhage, haematological cancer, infection, adrenal failure and major depressive disorders (see the articles listed in the Bibliography).

BIBLIOGRAPHY

Gordon, B. R., Parker, T. S., Levine, D. M., Saal, S. D., Wang, J. C., Sloan, B. J., et al. (1996) Low lipid concentrations in critical illness: implications for preventing and treating endotoxemia. *Critical Care Medicine*, 24(4), 584–589.

Gordon, B. R., Parker, T. S., Levine, D. M., Saal, S. D., Wang, J. C., Sloan, B. J., et al. (2001). Relationship of hypolipidemia to cytokine concentrations and outcomes in critically ill surgical patients. *Critical Care Medicine*, 29(8), 1563–1568.

Laing, E. (2020). Nutrition and metabolism. In Z. Tomkins (Ed.) *Applied anatomy and physiology – an interdisciplinary approach.* (1st ed.) (pp. 349–360). Chatswood, NSW: Elsevier.

On, W. H., Lim, Y. J., & Yap, K. (2020). Gastrointestinal system. In Z. Tomkins (Ed.) *Applied anatomy and physiology – an interdisciplinary approach.* (1st ed.) (pp. 329–348). Chatswood, NSW: Elsevier.

Papakostas, G. I., Iosifescu, D. V., Petersen, T., Hamill, S. K., Alpert, J. E., Nierenberg, A. A., et al. (2004). Serum cholesterol in the continuation phase of pharmacotherapy with fluoxetine in remitted major depressive disorder. *Journal of Clinical Psychopharmacology*, 24(4), 467–469.

Pugliese, L., Bernardini, I., Pacifico, N., Peverini, M., Damaskopoulou, E., Cataldi, S., et al. (2010). Severe hypocholesterolaemia is often neglected in haematological malignancies. *European Journal of Cancer*, 46(9), 1735–1743.

Tomkins, Z. (2020). Endocrine system. In Z. Tomkins (Ed.) *Applied anatomy and physiology – an interdisciplinary approach.* (1st ed.) (pp. 169–194). Chatswood, NSW: Elsevier.

CASE 8
Chronic stress and heart health

HISTORY

Karen was recently appointed as a new director of a business analytics unit. She was responsible for a team of seven people and for reaching a revenue target for the company. Karen is also a sole carer of two small children, aged 3 and 7 years. With exception of her sister, Karen has nobody else to turn to if she needs help in managing childcare and school needs.

Being new to the role, and in addition to her 40 hours a week job, Karen found she was working in the evenings once her children had gone to bed. Working long hours has left no time for relaxation, exercise or sufficient sleep. One afternoon, after experiencing a considerable amount of stress and anxiety following an unpleasant exchange with senior management, Karen felt her heart beating strongly, feeling like a flutter, and irregularly. She felt unwell and dizzy and needed to sit down.

This episode lasted for about 1 minute before she felt her heartbeat return to a more regular pace. Concerned that this may signal heart problems, and aware that her children depended on her wellbeing, Karen visited her local clinic. There she had an electrocardiogram (ECG) done, which did not show any abnormal changes. When asked about her family's history of heart disease, she revealed that, on her father's side, her grandfather and his brother had both passed away in their early sixties from a heart attack. She also revealed that, on her mother's side, the women were often diagnosed with chronic heart conditions but lived well into their nineties. When asked about her lifestyle and exercise, Karen shared the above information with her doctor.

Her doctor decided to order further tests to rule out hyperthyroidism and to refer her to a cardiologist. However, in the mean time, the doctor also suggested that the episode experienced may have been caused by severe levels of stress and together they discussed what options may be feasible.

QUESTIONS

1. Which division(s) of the autonomic nervous system control(s) the heart rate?

2. When considering Karen's presenting history, why was it important to do an ECG?

3. Why is the family history important in understanding an individual's risk of developing a cardiovascular condition?

4. Suggest why Karen's irregular heart rate may have been due to stress.

5. Why did the doctor want to rule out hyperthyroidism?

ANSWERS: CASE 8
Chronic stress and heart health

1. An increase in heart rate is regulated by the sympathetic nervous system, whereas a decrease in heart rate is regulated by the parasympathetic nervous system.

2. To understand why an ECG was performed, it is important to consider the conduction system of the heart. Karen's heartbeat starts in the sinoatrial node (SA node), where the pacemaker cells produce an electrical impulse that is then conducted directly towards the right atrium; the original path of conduction and associated structures are outlined in Figure 8.1. The impulse generated by the SA node is then conducted to the left atrium via the interatrial conducting bundle and fibres and to the atrioventricular (AV) node via the internodal bundle and fibres. Thereafter, the AV node directs the electrical impulse through the septum and the lateral walls of the right and left ventricles. This is possible because the conducting fibres branch from the AV node into right and left AV bundle branches, which further branch into subendocardial branches (also known as Purkinje fibres). Interruptions to this conduction pathway can occur at any point from the SA node to the Purkinje fibres. The ECG, a graphic record of the heart's electrical activity, helps detect whether there are irregularities along this pathway. This is of value as it can help indicate where the problem might have occurred along the conduction pathway and what part of the heart it may be affecting. Keep in mind, however, that an ECG trace does not give any information on heart contractility as it captures an event that precedes the contractility (i.e. electrical impulse that will later lead to contraction). It also does not detect coronary vessel blockages. In Karen's case, the ECG would help the diagnostic process as the clinicians seek to determine the cause of her increased heart rate and whether there may be an abnormality associated with that episode.

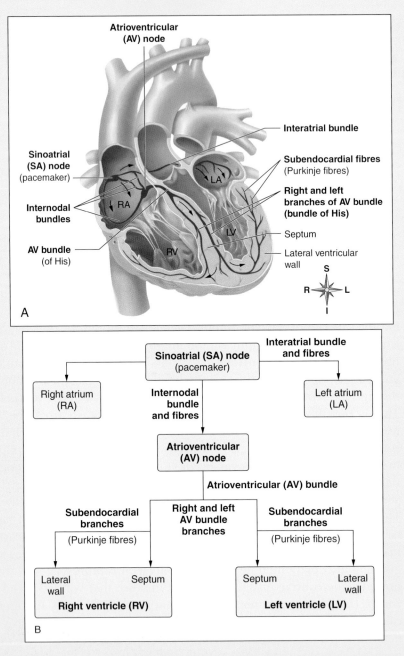

FIGURE 8.1 Conduction system of the heart. **A** Generation of the electrical impulse by the sinoatrial node and its path of travel through the heart. **B** Concept map of the origin and path of conduction.

3. A family history is important in understanding an individual's risk of developing a cardiovascular condition because heart disease is a polygenic condition, meaning that many genes play a role in its development, progression and outcome. Any person's risk of developing cardiovascular-related events can be estimated from the family's history, as each person is a product of their family genes. Understanding this risk helps an individual to make lifestyle adjustments to reduce their risk of developing a cardiovascular episode.

4. During her visit to her doctor, Karen spoke of an increased workload and more family commitments as a sole carer for her children. This means that she would be experiencing high levels of stress and may have anxiety about those pressures. Not being able to exercise (a protective factor), or get enough rest and sleep, means that her system is not getting enough time to recover. Stress has multiple physiological effects. One of them is prolonged activation of the fight or flight response, as demonstrated in Figure 8.2. Briefly, when stress occurs, the amygdala perceives a threat and sends a signal to the hypothalamus to stimulate several glands to release hormones so as to manage the physiological responses needed for responding to this threat. Through the sympathomedullary axis, the hypothalamus sends a signal to the adrenal medulla to release adrenaline (epinephrine). Adrenaline in turn acts on beta-1-adrenergic receptors to stimulate an increased heart rate and sweating, as well as increased glucose metabolism and oxygen uptake. It causes vasoconstriction, which increases peripheral vascular resistance, which impacts on blood pressure by increasing it. At the same time, the hypothalamus releases corticotropic hormone (CRH), which stimulates the anterior pituitary gland to release adrenocorticotropic hormone (ACTH). This hormone acts on the adrenal cortex gland to release the glucocorticoid cortisol and the mineralocorticoid aldosterone. Cortisol perpetuates the initial stress response. Aldosterone increases sodium and water reabsorption, which increases blood volume and, through this action, increases blood pressure. The hypothalamus will also stimulate the posterior pituitary gland to increase secretion of antidiuretic hormone (ADH), which increases diuresis (i.e. decreased water and urine retention) and so further contributes to increased blood volume, and so also increases blood pressure. Increased blood volume and increased blood pressure place an increased demand on the heart as it has to increase cardiac output (the volume of blood the heart pumps through the systemic circulation in a minute). As cardiac output is a product of stroke volume and the number of beats per minute (the heart rate), this increase in cardiac output will demand an increased heart rate.

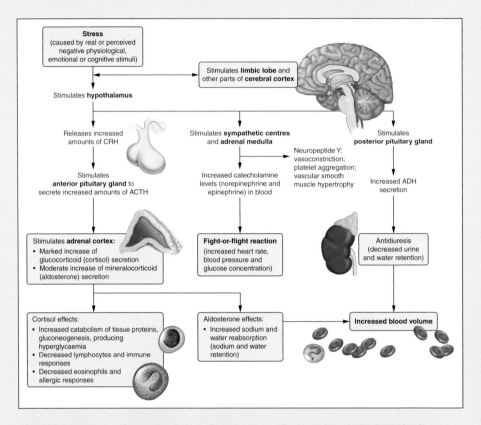

FIGURE 8.2 Effects of stress on fight or flight response. Prolonged cortisol release leads to these responses becoming chronic, meaning that the person is constantly in some form of fight or flight mode. ACTH = adrenocorticotropic hormone, ADH = antidiuretic hormone, CRH = corticotropic hormone.

In addition to the hormonal system, the autonomic nervous system also plays a role. During a stressful time, the sympathetic nervous system (SNS) also stimulates the adrenal medulla to release the catecholamine adrenaline (a hormone) and the sympathetic neurons to release the catecholamine noradrenaline (a neurotransmitter). Adrenaline and noradrenaline activate beta-1-adrenergic receptors on the SA node cells to increase the heart rate and conductivity and speed of the electrical impulses from the SA node to the AV node. This is evident in Karen's case as 'flutter'.

5. The doctor wanted to rule out the hyperthyroidism because rapid heartbeat, irregular heart beat and palpitations are common symptoms of hyperthyroidism – a condition where the thyroid gland produces an excessive amount of thyroid hormones. This in turn leads to heightened adrenergic stimulation and increased metabolic effects.

BIBLIOGRAPHY

Genetic Alliance; The New York-Mid-Atlantic Consortium for Genetic and Newborn Screening Services. (2009). *Understanding genetics: a New York, Mid-Atlantic guide for patients and health professionals.* Appendix B: Family history is important for your health. Washington, DC: Genetic Alliance, Jul 8. Available from: https://www.ncbi.nlm.nih.gov/books/NBK115560/?otool=iaumelblib.

Harris, P. R. (2016). The normal electrocardiogram: resting 12-lead and electrocardiogram monitoring in the hospital. *Critical Care Nursing Clinics of North America,* 28(3), 281–296.

McStacey, S. (2019) Recording a 12-lead electrocardiogram (ECG). *British Journal of Nursing,* 28(12), 756–760.

Nelson, S., & Tomkins, Z. (2020). Cardiovascular system. In Z. Tomkins (Ed.) *Applied anatomy and physiology – an interdisciplinary approach.* (1st ed.) (pp. 227–248). Chatswood, NSW: Elsevier.

Quan, K. J. (2019). Palpitation: extended electrocardiogram monitoring: which tests to use and when. *Medical Clinics of North America,* 103(5), 785–791.

Tomkins, Z. (2020). Endocrine system. In Z. Tomkins (Ed.) *Applied anatomy and physiology – an interdisciplinary approach.* (1st ed.) (pp. 169–194). Chatswood, NSW: Elsevier.

Tomkins, Z. (2020). Genes and genomics. In Z. Tomkins (Ed.) *Applied anatomy and physiology – an interdisciplinary approach.* (1st ed.) (pp. 29–52). Chatswood, NSW: Elsevier.

CASE 9
Significant blood loss due to internal injuries

HISTORY

A 23-year-old man, Simon, was involved in a motor vehicle accident in which a car had gone through a red light and hit his car on the left side. Simon was travelling at 80 kilometres an hour, as was the car that hit him. His car had rolled several times before it stopped. The driver of the other car suffered only minor injuries and was able to call an ambulance and a fire engine to the scene. Simon was conscious and coherent but in significant pain. He had laboured breathing and extensive bruising and abrasions on his right side. Prior to the accident, Simon had no previous health issues and no known allergies.

At the site of the accident, once the fire brigade extricated him, it was recorded that Simon was in pain (pain score 8.5/10), peripherally cool and diaphoretic with a blood pressure of 110/75 mmHg, pulse of 110 beats per minute and respiratory rate of 24 breaths per minute. His Glasgow Coma Scale score was 13. The paramedic documented that Simon was using his accessory muscles of respiration and supporting his right-side chest with his hands. Concerns were raised about possible internal injuries and fractured ribs. By the time Simon was transported into the emergency department, his condition had deteriorated so that his pulse was 130 beats per minute, his systolic blood pressure was 90/55 mmHg, his respiratory rate was 29 breaths per minute and he was semiconscious with a Glasgow Coma Scale score of 11, with his pupils equal and reactive. There was reduced air entry and coarse crackles on both sides of his chest.

QUESTIONS

1. Why might Simon have been experiencing difficulties with his breathing at the scene of the accident?

2. Describe how difficulties in breathing may affect gas exchange in the lungs.

3. If Simon has internal bleeding, detail how acute blood loss would affect oxygen transport to Simon's tissues.

4. In the absence of an adequate blood oxygen supply to the tissue, suggest how this would affect blood pH and haemoglobin affinity for oxygen.

5. Use a concept map to illustrate how the cardiac, neuronal, endocrine and renal systems cooperate to maintain blood pressure in the early stages of internal blood loss (haemorrhage).

6. Considering that the Glasgow Coma Scale measures eye opening, verbal response and motor response, what is the significance of the Glasgow Coma Scale score decreasing from 13 to 11 in Simon's case?

ANSWERS: CASE 9
Significant blood loss due to internal injuries

1. Difficulties with breathing are due to Simon bruising and/or fracturing his ribs. If the ribs are fractured, it is possible that the sharp end of the fractured rib has punctured the lung pleura and the lung, leading to formation of pneumothorax (air in the lung), haemothorax (blood in the lung) and/or haemopneumothorax (air and blood in the lung) (Figure 9.1). These injuries lead to air entering the space between the chest wall and the lung (pleural cavity) and loss of intrapleural negative pressure, causing

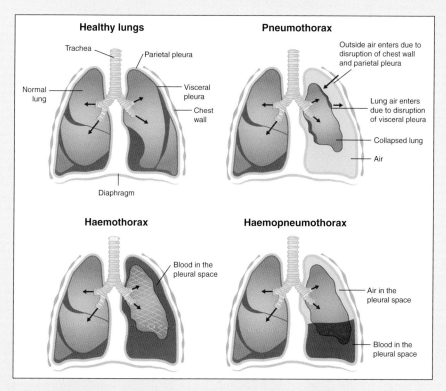

FIGURE 9.1 Healthy lungs and changes associated with rib injuries that lead to difficulties with breathing.
Source: https://depositphotos.com/275452090/stock-illustration-human-lungs-with-pneumothorax-hemothorax.html

the affected lung to collapse. This also causes decreased vital lung capacity and a decrease in the arterial oxygen pressure (P_aO_2). Fractured ribs and associated bruising cause pain. To minimise the experience of pain, Simon may try to control his rate and depth of breathing, so limiting rib cage movement and causing reduced alveolar ventilation.

2. To understand the effect of lung injury in Simon's case on gas exchange, consider the normal process of inspiration. During normal inspiration, oxygen diffuses into the blood through the respiratory membrane, while carbon dioxide diffuses from the blood into the lung alveoli. Once in the blood, 98.5% of the oxygen binds to haemoglobin to form oxyhaemoglobin, whereas 1.5% will travel dissolved in the blood. As dissolved oxygen diffuses out of arterial blood, due to pressure gradient difference towards cells, blood P_aO_2 decreases. This accelerates oxyhaemoglobin dissociation, releasing more oxygen to plasma for diffusion into the cells. When carbon dioxide, which is produced during cell catabolism, diffuses from the cell into the blood, most of it is converted to carbaminohaemoglobin and hydrogen ions, or bicarbonate and hydrogen ions. This increase in PCO_2 favours oxygen dissociation from haemoglobin, decreases the affinity between haemoglobin and oxygen (or right shift in oxygen-haemoglobin association curve) and increases CO_2 association with haemoglobin to form carbaminohaemoglobin.

3. In Simon's case, the fracture and pain cause a loss of capacity to increase the anterior–posterior dimensions of his thorax, and therefore a decreased capacity to expand his thoracic cage; the loss of pleural space integrity and a collapsed lung result in a loss of capacity to inhale and exhale as needed and a decreased vital capacity (Figure 9.2). This leads to reduced alveolar ventilation and reduced alveolar PO_2, and therefore reduced blood O_2 diffusion and so less O_2 is available to bind to haemoglobin to form oxyhaemoglobin in the erythrocytes. At the same time, CO_2 from metabolism cannot be cleared effectively from the lung, leading to its build-up in alveoli but also in the bloodstream, where it leads to increased blood pH and increased affinity of haemoglobin molecules to bind more CO_2 to form carboxyhaemoglobin.

4. In Simon's case, as a result of blood loss his blood contains fewer erythrocytes and therefore there is less haemoglobin available to carry oxygen to the tissues (each haemoglobin molecule binds four oxygen atoms). This leads to hypoxaemia and then tissue hypoxia and ischaemic injury.

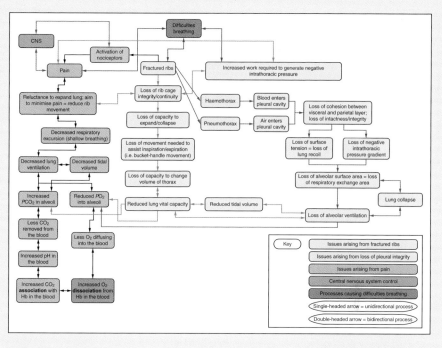

FIGURE 9.2. Effect of impaired inhalation and exhalation on gas exchange in the lungs.

5. Lack of an adequate oxygen supply from the lung alveoli to the blood leads to a decrease in pH, while haemoglobin affinity for oxygen will decrease. This is because tissue metabolism continues to produce CO_2 in the presence of a chronic reduction in O_2 supply. When CO_2 enters the blood, it is converted to carbaminohaemoglobin and hydrogen ions (H^+), or to bicarbonate and H^+. Hence increasing the CO_2 content of the blood also increases the blood H^+ concentration, leading to acidaemia or a drop in pH in the blood. Normally, during cell catabolism, oxygen is used for aerobic respiration to produce adenosine triphosphate, an energy source within the cell, and CO_2, a metabolic waste product. In Simon's case, hypoxia causes a switch to anaerobic metabolism and so more lactic acid is produced, hence contributing to a further decrease in pH levels. This will cause a significant right shift in the oxyhaemoglobin dissociation curve (Figure 9.3), whereby oxygen will have a lower affinity for haemoglobin and erythrocytes will release O_2 more readily. This has a twofold impact: (i) more O_2 is released to the cells and (ii) at lung level, less O_2 binds to erythrocytes, meaning that over time less and less

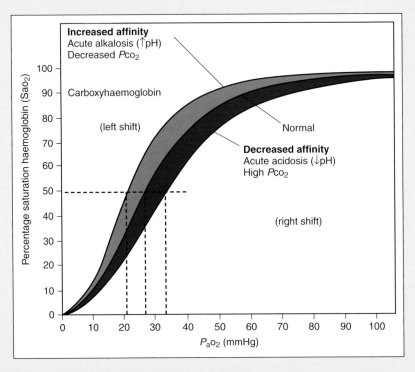

FIGURE 9.3 Oxyhaemoglobin dissociation curve representing changes in haemoglobin saturation (S_aO_2) with changes in the partial pressure of oxygen (P_aO_2). The flat segment of the curve at the top of the graph represents the arterial or association portion where oxygen is bound to haemoglobin in the lungs. This portion of the curve is flat because partial pressure changes of oxygen between 60 and 100 mmHg do not significantly alter the percentage saturation of haemoglobin with oxygen and allow adequate haemoglobin saturation at a variety of altitudes. The steep part of the oxyhaemoglobin dissociation curve represents the rapid dissociation of oxygen from haemoglobin that occurs in the tissues. During this phase, there is rapid diffusion of oxygen from the blood into tissue cells. The P_{50} is the P_aO_2 at which haemoglobin is 50% saturated (normally 26.6 mmHg). A lower than normal P_{50} represents increased affinity of haemoglobin for O_2; a high P_{50} is seen with decreased affinity. With a decrease in pH (acidosis), high CO_2 levels will favour decreased affinity of haemoglobin for oxygen.
Modified from Figure 35.16 from McCance, K. L., & Huether, S. E. (2019). *Pathophysiology: the biologic basis for disease in adults and children* (8th ed). St Louis, MO: Elsevier, p. 1157.

O_2 would be delivered to the tissue if the acidosis is unresolved. The opposite is true for CO_2, which would bind more easily to haemoglobin at tissue level, but it would be harder to release it in the lung, where alveolar CO_2 may be increased. For Simon this will be manifested in a reduced blood oxygen saturation level and an increased respiratory rate. The concept map (Figure 9.4) captures these events.

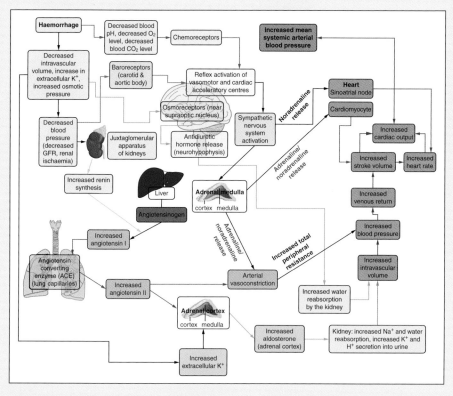

FIGURE 9.4 A concept map of integrated responses from the renal, cardiac, neuronal and endocrine systems to maintain blood pressure in early stages of haemorrhage.

6. Reduced intravascular volume will impact on the blood pressure needed for perfusion of the brain tissue and maintenance of neuronal function. As the blood volume to the brain decreases, so too any functions that the brain controls start to shut down so that eventually only those required for survival are sustained (Figure 9.4). In Simon's case, the function that is changing now is the level of consciousness and how this impacts on his verbal and motor responses, as measured by the Glasgow Coma Scale.

BIBLIOGRAPHY

Bridge, N., & Tomkins, Z. (2020). Respiratory system. In Z. Tomkins (Ed.) *Applied anatomy and physiology – an interdisciplinary approach.* (1st ed.) (pp. 305–328). Chatswood, NSW: Elsevier.

Chopra, S., Baby, C., & Jacob, J. J. (2011). Neuro-endocrine regulation of blood pressure. *Indian Journal of Endocrinology and Metabolism*, 15(Suppl4), S281–S288. doi: 10.4103/2230-8210.86860.

Glasgow Coma Scale. Available at https://www.glasgowcomascale.org/.

Montayre, J., Macdiarmid, R., McDonald, E. M., & Saravanakumar, P. (2020). Urinary system. In Z. Tomkins (Ed.) *Applied anatomy and physiology – an interdisciplinary approach.* (1st ed.) (pp. 361–382). Chatswood, NSW: Elsevier.

Nelson, S., & Tomkins, Z. (2020). Cardiovascular system. In Z. Tomkins (Ed.) *Applied anatomy and physiology – an interdisciplinary approach.* (1st ed.) (pp. 227–248). Chatswood, NSW: Elsevier.

Shahoud, J. S., & Aeddula, N. R. (2020). Physiology, arterial pressure regulation. In *StatPearls* [Internet]. Treasure Island, FL: StatPearls Publishing. Available from: https://www.ncbi.nlm.nih.gov/books/NBK538509/.

Tulaimat, A., & Trick, W. E. (2017). DiapHRaGM: a mnemonic to describe the work of breathing in patients with respiratory failure. *PloS One*, 12(7), e0179641. doi: 10.1371/journal.pone.0179641.

Tulaimat, A., Patel, A., Wisniewski, M., & Gueret, R. (2016). The validity and reliability of the clinical assessment of increased work of breathing in acutely ill patients. *Journal of Critical Care*, 34, 111–115. doi: 10.1016/j.jcrc.2016.04.013.

Tomkins, Z. (2020). Endocrine system. In Z. Tomkins (Ed.) *Applied anatomy and physiology – an interdisciplinary approach.* (1st ed.) (pp. 169–194). Chatswood, NSW: Elsevier.

CASE 10
Flu vaccination

HISTORY

David is a third year Bachelor of Nursing student and is currently attending a clinical placement in the aged care centre. Over the last 4 days, three staff members have called in sick because they had flu-like symptoms. David is worried that, if he develops flu himself, he may not complete his clinical placement on time, which may impact on his course progression. He is also very concerned about how the illness of three staff members may impact on the elderly in the aged care residence. He expressed these concerns during a debriefing session with other students and his Clinical Nurse Educator (CNE), Peter.

QUESTIONS

1. Peter asks David whether he has been in contact with anyone who may have the flu. Explain why this information is of significance in terms of transmission of an influenza virus from person to person.

2. Describe what may occur when an influenza virus enters the body.

3. What immune responses aimed at combating the influenza virus are most likely to take place?

4. Peter also asks David whether he has had an annual flu shot. Explain why flu shots have a valuable role in protecting David from developing flu, and the impact on elderly residents in his care.

5. Discuss the role of immunological memory in protecting David from subsequent exposure to the same strain of this infectious agent.

ANSWERS: CASE 10
Flu vaccination

1. Flu is caused by influenza virus (serotypes A, B and C, of which A and B cause respiratory illness). The virus is transmitted: (1) by direct contact with infected individuals via droplets, (2) by contact with contaminated objects onto which the droplets have fallen, and (3) by inhalation of virus-laden aerosol particles (Figure 10.1). Objects that are contaminated by microorganisms or viruses are known as fomites and include items such as doorknobs, curtains, surfaces or a patient's personal objects (including toys).

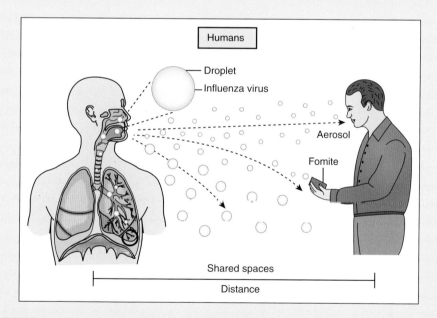

FIGURE 10.1 Mode of transmission of influenza virus.

Previous contact with someone who has had flu might increase David's chances of being exposed to the virus.

2. When it enters the body, the influenza virus must overcome three lines of defence. The first line (innate immunity) comprises the epithelial

cells in the upper respiratory airways, lungs and their membrane barriers (and their secretions), and the body's normal microbial flora (Figure 10.2). The second line of defence (innate immunity) comprises phagocytosis, inflammation, cytokines and antimicrobial proteins. These defences have the important characteristic of rapid response – that is, they are activated within minutes to hours of a microbe entering the tissues. Acquired or adaptive immunity refers to the body's third line of defence; it involves a mechanism that recognises specific threatening agents (foreign substances, termed antigens, and abnormal or infected cells) and then adapts by inducing a specific immune response against these microorganisms.

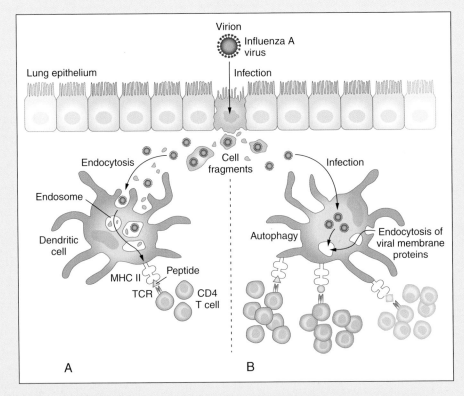

FIGURE 10.2 Mechanisms of influenza A virus infecting lung epithelial cells. **A** The fragments of dead, infected epithelial cell are ingested by the antigen-presenting cells (such as dendritic cells) during the process called endocytosis. **B** Alternatively, virion particles released by the infected cells actively infect antigen-presenting cells (macrophages, dendritic cells), and their fragments are presented to the naïve T cells (CD4+ T cells) via the MHC II molecule. This will then lead to activation of cell-mediated and antibody-mediated immunity (previously shown in Figure 1.6).

3. The rate and strength of response to influenza virus depend on whether the person has been previously immunised against the infectious strain of the virus. In the absence of immunisation, the defence will predominantly involve adaptive immunity, with activation of T-cell-mediated responses, where cytotoxic T cells destroy the infected cells; T-helper cells will also induce flu-specific B cells to undergo clonal selection and fine tuning to develop antibody-mediated responses to flu virus. A small proportion of the virus-specific T and B cells will differentiate to form a memory of their response to that specific strain of influenza virus and will remain in the individual's tissues long after the infection has been cleared (see Figure 1.6).

4. The vaccination status indicates the degree of protection David may have during the flu season (i.e. the influenza vaccine may decrease the likelihood of developing flu). As influenza vaccination contains strains of dead or attenuated influenza viruses (pathogens), they will stimulate David's body to develop antibodies (through B-cell clonal selection and cellular immunity), which would protect him from the actual virus once the exposure occurs or result in a significantly lighter infection that would be easier to overcome. This is a type of artificial acquired immunity. Until recently it was thought that, by protecting himself, he is also participating in herd immunity, which protects the elderly in his care. (See the two Cochrane reviews by Demicheli et al in the Bibliography, which discuss this in great depth.)

5. Re-exposure to the same antigen would lead to activation of memory B and T cells. Through clonal replication of those cells, an immune response would be deployed much earlier, leading to a faster combative response and quicker recovery.

BIBLIOGRAPHY

Abdelkader, A., & Barbagallo, M. S. (2020). Immune system. In Z. Tomkins (Ed.) *Applied anatomy and physiology – an interdisciplinary approach*. (1st ed.) (pp. 265–278). Chatswood, NSW: Elsevier.

Demicheli, V., Jefferson, T., Di Pietrantonj, C., Ferroni, E., Thorning, S., Thomas, R. E., et al. (2018). Vaccines for preventing influenza in the elderly. *Cochrane Database of Systematic Reviews*, 2, CD004876. doi: 10.1002/14651858.CD004876.pub4.

Demicheli, V., Jefferson, T., Ferroni, E., Rivetti, A., & Di Pietrantonj, C. (2018). Vaccines for preventing influenza in healthy adults. *Cochrane Database of Systematic Reviews*, 2, CD001269. doi: 10.1002/14651858.CD001269.pub6.

Ghebrehewet, S., MacPherson, P., & Ho, A. (2016). Influenza. *British Medical Journal*, 355, i6258.

Grohskopf, L. A., Alyanak, E., Broder, K. R., Walter, E. B., Fry, A. M., & Jernigan, D. B. (2019). Prevention and control of seasonal influenza with vaccines: recommendations of the Advisory Committee on Immunization Practices – United States, 2019–20 influenza season. *Morbidity and Mortality Weekly Report Recommendations and Reports*, 68(RR-3), 1–21. doi: http://dx.doi.org/10.15585/mmwr.rr6803a1.

Jefferson, T., Rivetti, A., Di Pietrantonj, C., & Demicheli, V. (2018). Vaccines for preventing influenza in healthy children. *Cochrane Database of Systematic Reviews*, 2, CD004879. doi: 10.1002/14651858.CD004879.pub5.

Mintern, J., & Villadangos, J. (2015). Antigen-presenting cells look within during influenza infection. *Nature Medicine*, 21, 1123–1125. doi: 10.1038/nm.3971.

Tomkins, Z. (2020). Acute inflammation. In Z. Tomkins (Ed.) *Applied anatomy and physiology – an interdisciplinary approach.* (1st ed.) (pp. 279–304). Chatswood, NSW: Elsevier.

Treanor J. (2016). Influenza vaccination. *New England Journal of Medicine*, 375(13), 1261–1268.

CASE 11
A teenager with an allergic reaction to peanuts

HISTORY

A 15-year-old schoolgirl was admitted to the emergency department following an allergic reaction to peanuts while on a school excursion. This is not the first time that she has been treated at the emergency department. Previously, she was admitted at 7 years of age, after she accidentally ate food containing traces of peanuts at the local restaurant and experienced tightness in her throat and difficulty breathing. This occurred about 5 minutes after she had ingested the contaminated food. During her current presentation to the emergency department, she had marked angioedema of her face, lips and tongue, severe throat constriction and was vomiting. According to her schoolteacher, the girl had developed angioedema of her lips and tongue and difficulty in breathing and had reported feeling light-headed within minutes. Her teacher had administered an EpiPen injection while waiting for paramedics to arrive.

QUESTIONS

1. Explain the immune response associated with the primary exposure to peanut allergen.

2. Discuss the immune response associated with secondary and subsequent exposures to nut allergen and explain why subsequent exposures resulted in faster response to the allergen.

3. Why did the teacher administer an EpiPen injection?

ANSWERS: CASE 11
A teenager with an allergic reaction to peanuts

1. Peanut allergy is an IgE-mediated and cell-mediated response to peanut allergen. It is important to recognise that the immune response to peanut allergy will be determined by the type of allergen encountered, as the peanuts have 12 recognised allergens that can induce an immune response. Broadly, these can be grouped into major and minor allergens. When IgE-secreting B cells encounter peanut allergen, they secrete IgE antibodies that strongly bind to several forms of peanut allergen.

2. During the first exposure (Figure 11.1), the peanut allergen is most likely to be introduced via a subset of intestinal epithelial cells called M cells. These cells transfer the antigen to submucosa, where the allergen is ingested by the antigen-presenting cells (such as dendritic cells) and processed into peptide fragment. The peptide fragment is expressed on the cell surface of the antigen-presenting cell by MHC class II molecules. When a MHC class II molecule interacts with the T-cell receptor on the naïve T-helper cell, the T-helper cell becomes primed and activated. This precipitates an antibody-mediated response as well as a cell-mediated response. For example, T-helper cells secrete cytokines, which, during sensitisation process, act on IgE-secreting B cells resulting in secretion of more IgE antibodies. These antibodies bind to peanut allergen in an attempt to eliminate it. From a cellular-mediated response, T-helper-2 (T_H2) cells secrete other cytokines (such as interleukins 2, 5 and 13) and help IgE-secreting B cells to produce more peanut-specific IgE. Using the stem part of IgE, the IgE molecule binds to mast cells and basophils via surface IgE receptors. Memory T cells, memory B cells and plasma B cells will also form, which will cause the immune system to react faster on subsequent occasions.

    On subsequent exposure to peanut allergens, the peanut protein binds to specific IgE antibody on the mast cells and basophils. This reaction causes degranulation of mast cells and basophils, which is characterised by a release of histamine, prostaglandins, leukotrienes and other cytokines, which collectively act as inflammatory agents (see Figure 11.1). Some of those cytokines also cause eosinophils to be recruited to the site of allergen exposure. Plasma B cells and memory B cells will also become re-activated to add to the response to the allergen, which further potentiates the inflammatory response. Part of the inflammatory response is hyperpermeable (leaky) blood vessels, which is clinically evident as angioedema of the lips and tongue, and which may then directly lead to difficulty in breathing and reported light-headedness.

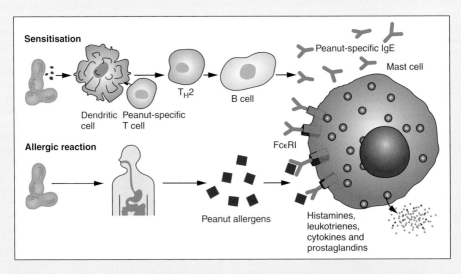

FIGURE 11.1 Sensitisation and allergic reactions to peanut allergens. Dendritic cells in the skin pick up peanut allergens and present them to peanut allergen-specific T-helper-2 (T_H2) cells, which in turn present them to B cells. Interaction between allergen-specific T_H2 cells and B cells solicits help from T_H2 cells for B-cell proliferation, somatic hypermutation and affinity maturation, class switching to IgE and plasma cell differentiation. Allergen-specific IgE secreted by plasma cells binds to resident mast cells in the gut, so the ingestion of peanuts triggers an allergic reaction.

3. The purpose of administering the EpiPen, which contains adrenaline, is to reverse the anaphylactic response, which is a multisystem allergic reaction. Adrenaline can act via three different adrenergic receptors, with each receptor pathway regulating a different outcome. It is a potent vasoconstrictor (acting through alpha-1-adrenergic receptors expressed by vascular smooth muscle cells), meaning that it reverses the peripheral vasodilation and therefore increases peripheral resistance while preventing peripheral oedema, leading to increased blood pressure, increased coronary blood flow, myocardial contractility

and cardiac output and suppressed additional release of inflammatory mediators from mast cells and basophils. Adrenaline also acts as a bronchodilator, which reduces resistance to air flow into and out of the lung and decreases the effort of breathing.

BIBLIOGRAPHY

Abdelkader, A., & Barbagallo, M. S. (2020). Immune system. In Z. Tomkins (Ed.) *Applied anatomy and physiology – an interdisciplinary approach.* (1st ed.) (pp. 265–278). Chatswood, NSW: Elsevier.

Burks, A. W. (2008). Peanut allergy. *The Lancet,* 371(9623), 1538–1546,

Costa C., Coimbra A., Vítor A., Aguiar R., Ferreira A. L., & Todo-Bom A. (2020). Food allergy – from food avoidance to active treatment. *Scandinavian Journal of Immunology,* 91(1), e12824.

Croote, D., Darmanis, S., Nadeau, K. C., & Quake, S. R. (2018). High-affinity allergen-specific human antibodies cloned from single IgE B cell transcriptomes. *Science,* 362(6420), 1306–1309.

Mueller, G. A., Maleki, S. J., & Pedersen, L. C. (2014). The molecular basis of peanut allergy. *Current Allergy and Asthma Reports,* 14(5), 429. doi: 10.1007/s11882-014-0429-5.

Nelson, S., & Tomkins, Z. (2020). Cardiovascular system. In Z. Tomkins (Ed.) *Applied anatomy and physiology – an interdisciplinary approach.* (1st ed.) (pp. 227–248). Chatswood, NSW: Elsevier.

Simons, F. E. R., Ardusso, L. R., Bilò, M. B., Cardona, V., Ebisawa, M., El-Gamal, Y. M., et al. (2014) International consensus on (ICON) anaphylaxis. *World Allergy Organization Journal,* 7, 1–19.

Yap, K. (2020). Nervous system. In Z. Tomkins (Ed.) *Applied anatomy and physiology – an interdisciplinary approach.* (1st ed.) (pp. 113–134). Chatswood, NSW: Elsevier.

Yu, W., Freeland, D., & Nadeau, K. C. (2016). Food allergy: immune mechanisms, diagnosis and immunotherapy. *Nature Reviews. Immunology,* 16(12), 751–765.

CASE 12
A cyclist with a heart attack

HISTORY

Joe is an avid cyclist and, on most days, he rides 75 kilometres a day to work and back home. He leads a healthy lifestyle, is not a smoker and he abstains from alcohol. This morning Joe got out of bed as usual and was enjoying his breakfast when he felt a crushing pain in his chest. Recognising that Joe may be having a heart attack, his partner, John, phoned the ambulance. Paramedics did an electrocardiogram (ECG) while in the emergency department, blood tests were ordered for cardiac troponin I and an urgent angiogram (a test that visualises coronary vessels in real time) was performed. The cardiac troponin I level indicated that a substantial damage has occurred to the myocardium, while the angiogram indicated that a clot has caused an 80% occlusion of the left descending coronary artery.

QUESTIONS

1. Prior to Joe's heart attack, discuss how the coronary arteries supply oxygen and nutrients needed for cardiac muscle function.

2. If the clot causing Joe's heart attack has blocked the left descending coronary artery, which part of the heart/cardiac muscle would be affected by this blockage and would this cause a major or a minor heart attack?

3. Explain why Joe feels chest pain if there is an impairment of the blood flow to his heart.

4. Discuss why an electrocardiogram was required in this case and what do you expect it may show, considering that the left descending artery was blocked?

5. What is troponin I, what is its function and why would elevated blood levels of troponin I indicate heart damage?

ANSWERS: CASE 12
A cyclist with a heart attack

1. Two coronary arteries, the left and right coronary arteries, originate from the left side of the heart from the left and aortic sinuses (Figure 12.1A). These sinuses are located within the aorta behind the right and left flaps of the aortic valve. The left and right coronary arteries fill with blood when the heart is relaxed as this allows the back-flow of the blood filling the valve pockets and movement into the coronary arteries. The left coronary artery branches into the left anterior descending artery and the left circumflex artery. The right coronary artery branches to form the right marginal artery. In general, the left anterior descending artery and its branches supply the interventricular septum, the anterior, lateral and apical walls of the left ventricle, most of the right and left bundle branches, and the anterior papillary muscle of the bicuspid valve, which is in the left ventricle. It also provides collateral circulation to the anterior right ventricle, the posterior part of the interventricular septum and the posterior descending artery. Blood enters the myocardial capillaries then trains into the thespian veins. These merge into larger coronary veins, which then merge to drain into

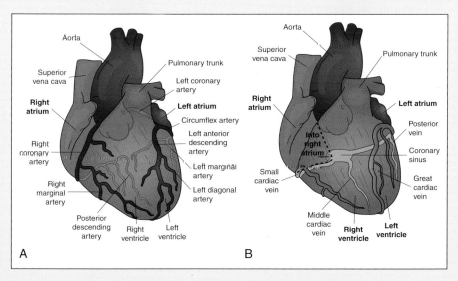

FIGURE 12.1 Distribution of (**A**) coronary arteries and (**B**) coronary veins.

the coronary sinus (Figure 12.1B). This main vein of the heart drains into the right atrium at a site approximately located between the right atrioventricular (AV) opening and the inferior vena cava opening.

2. Near occlusion of the left descending coronary artery would significantly reduce blood supply to all its branches leading to very reduced blood flow to the interventricular septum, the anterior, lateral and apical walls of the left ventricle, most of the right and left bundle branches, the anterior papillary muscle of the bicuspid valve (in the left ventricle) and collaterally the anterior right ventricle, the posterior part of the interventricular septum and the posterior descending artery. This would cause substantial damage to the myocardium, which is clinically demonstrated as crushing chest pain and would be a major heart attack.

3. Decreased oxygen supply to the cardiomyocytes causes cellular stress and damage. Where oxygen has been depleted and the cell has subsequently died, a process of coagulative necrosis and inflammation will take place. This leads to reduced levels of adenosine triphosphate (ATP), the energy source needed by the cardiomyocytes to perform their function (Figure 12.2). It also leads to localised increase of CO_2 and metabolic products. Damage tends to start at the endocardium level first, as this is most distal to the blocked arterial blood supply, then spreads inwards through the myocardium. Damage arising from the reduced oxygen supply (hypoxaemia) causes ischaemia (reduced tissue oxygen levels). Combined with the damaging impact of accumulating metabolic products and cellular membrane changes, this causes a release of pro-inflammatory cytokines, including prostaglandins, which will stimulate nociceptors, which in turn carry the signal over to neuronal networks that register this as pain. Sympathetic afferent cardiac neurons are also activated and signal to the central nervous system that pain response is appropriate.

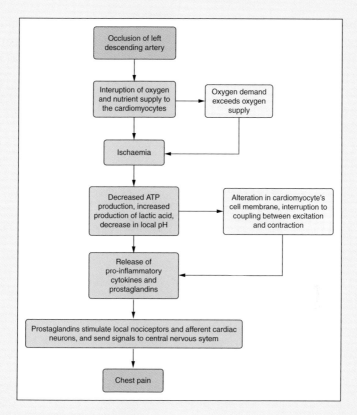

FIGURE 12.2 Cellular changes leading to stimulation of pain sensation during myocardial infarction.

4. Electrical impulses are spontaneously generated in the sinoatrial (SA) node, from where they spread across the atrial myocardium, causing contraction, and to the atrioventricular (AV) node (Figure 12.3A). Here there is a slight delay in conduction, which facilitates ventricular filling. From the AV node, impulses are conducted to the bundle of His, then to the right and left bundle branches and finally to the Purkinje fibres, where the impulses spread into the ventricular myocardium, causing contraction. An ECG (Figure 12.3B) provides a record of:

a. when the atrium is depolarised in response to SA node triggering (P wave);

b. the delay at the AV node to permit filling of the ventricles (PR interval);

c. the depolarisation of the ventricles, which initiates the main pumping contraction (QRS interval);

d. the beginning of ventricular repolarisation (ST segment); and

e. the ventricular repolarisation (T wave).

As the damage occurs to the cardiomyocytes and their cellular membrane becomes impaired, this will automatically affect the conduction of the electrical impulse in one or more of these sites. Hence, an ECG will be able to detect where the interruptions have occurred and the extent of those interruptions. Indirectly, it will be able to indicate the exact area where the myocardium is damaged.

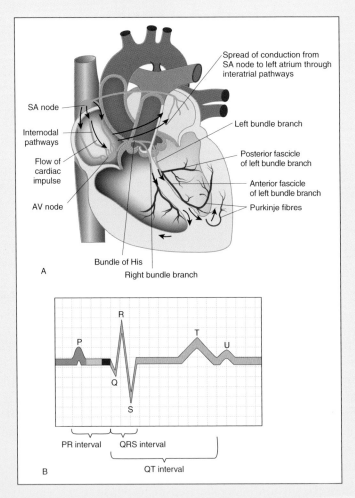

FIGURE 12.3 **A** Normal conduction system of the heart. **B** Its corresponding ECG pattern.

5. Troponin I is a structural element of the cardiac muscle; together with cardiac troponin C and cardiac troponin T, it comprises part of the thin filament that is complexed to actin in the cardiac muscle (Figure 12.4A). Collectively the troponin–actin complex

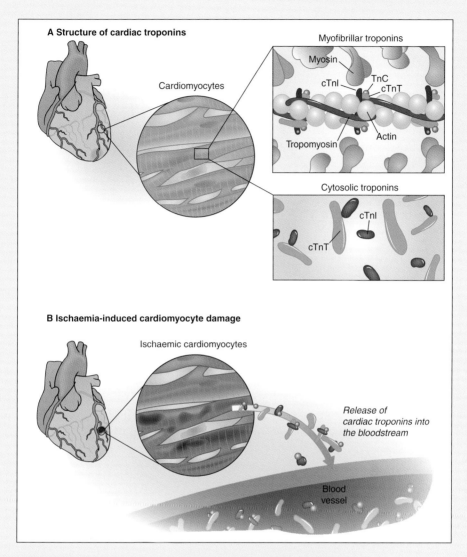

FIGURE 12.4 A Cardiac myocyte is composed of bundles of myofibrils that contain myofilaments. Each myofibril has a thick and a thin filament. The thick filament is composed of myosin. The thin filament is composed of actin and tropomysin. Each tropomysin contains troponin complex distributed at regular intervals. The troponin complex is made up of three subunits: troponin T, which attaches to the tropomysin, troponin C, which is a binding site for Ca^{2+} during excitation–contraction couplings, and troponin I, which inhibits the myosin-binding site on the actin filament. **B** Release of cardiac troponins following ischaemia-induced cardiac injury, such as that caused by the clot occlusion, leads to their presence in systemic circulation, so enabling their detection and measurement over a time period. TnC = troponin C, cTnI = cardiac troponin I, cTnT = cardiac troponin T.

is responsible for the cardiomyocyte contractile cycle. When the damage occurs, troponin is released into the circulation, where it is detectable as the marker of myocardial damage (Figure 12.4B). In Joe's case, troponin I would be indicative of the extent of the myocardial damage but would not be indicative of the location of where the damage occurred and it would not be diagnostic of a myocardial infarction, as troponin I is also often elevated in other cardiac conditions such as angina pectoris or atrial fibrillation.

BIBLIOGRAPHY

Cardiac muscle tissue. Lumen Boundless Anatomy and Physiology. From https://courses.lumenlearning.com/boundless-ap/chapter/cardiac-muscle-tissue/.

de Lemos, J. A. (2013). Increasingly sensitive assays for cardiac troponins: a review. *Journal of the American Medical Association*, 309(21), 2262–2269.

Leach, A., & Fisher, M. (2013). Myocardial ischaemia and cardiac pain – a mysterious relationship. *British Journal of Pain*, 7(1), 23–30.

Nelson, S., & Tomkins, Z. (2020). Cardiovascular system. In Z. Tomkins (Ed.) *Applied anatomy and physiology – an interdisciplinary approach*. (1st ed.) (pp. 227–248). Chatswood, NSW: Elsevier.

Shah, A., Sandoval, Y., Noaman, A., Sexter, A., Vaswani, A., Smith, S. W., et al. (2017). Patient selection for high sensitivity cardiac troponin testing and diagnosis of myocardial infarction: prospective cohort study. BMJ (Clinical research ed.), 359, j4788.

Tomkins, Z. (2020). Cellular response to injury. In Z. Tomkins (Ed.) *Applied anatomy and physiology – an interdisciplinary approach*. (1st ed.) (pp. 1–28). Chatswood, NSW: Elsevier.

CASE 13

Age-related changes in the respiratory, cardiovascular and musculoskeletal systems

HISTORY

David is 90 years old. He lives with his daughter, Gemma and her family of three children. David has no health problems and enjoys the company of his grandchildren. The only issue that bothers David is that he is no longer able to climb stairs as easily as he used to. By the time he has climbed to the first floor, he feels short of breath. However, he is not keen to stop climbing stairs as he sees this as his daily exercise.

QUESTIONS

1. What age-related changes would you expect to see in David's lungs, heart and musculoskeletal system?

2. Describe how these changes would lead to David feeling breathless when he climbs flights of stairs.

3. Why may age-related changes in the lungs impact on the function of the skeletal muscles, and could these changes be the reason why David may also feel muscle stiffness?

ANSWERS: CASE 13
Age-related changes in the respiratory, cardiovascular and musculoskeletal systems

1. As a human being ages, there is a change in the capacity to renew the cells lining tissues and organs, in deposition of the extracellular matrix and in the production of cytokines and growth factors that aid many functions in the body. In the lung, there is a decrease in elasticity of the alveoli, leading to reduced elastic recoil (Figure 13.1). The formation and movement of cilia and mucus production are also reduced. There is a decrease in the volume of the thoracic cavity and lung volume, as well as a reduced capacity of the muscles that aid respiration (such as the diaphragm, and abdominal and intercostal muscles). The decrease in lung ventilation and the increase in residual lung volume lead to reduced diffusion of oxygen into the blood. David's posture will also change as he ages, which will impact how he expands his lungs. Similarly, the cough reflex is decreased.

David's heart will start to accumulate lipofuscin, a pigment associated with ageing. His heart valves and larger arteries will become thicker and become stiffer, which will impact on how the blood flows through his cardiovascular system. His sinoatrial node may not be able to generate as many impulses when the heart needs to increase its work as the pacemaker cells have decreased in number; some of those impulses may also be irregular. Depending on his diet, he may have an increase in fatty deposits in his arteries, which may also impact the supply of oxygen and nutrition to his heart.

David's musculoskeletal system will show a loss of bone density, and of cartilage, decreased joint elasticity and decreased bone mass and volume in the intervertebral discs, which leads to posture changes. His rib cage will undergo structural changes that will make it more rigid. The muscles become hypotrophic and some are replaced with fat cells. Many of these changes are also linked to age-related changes in hormone concentrations – for example, those of testosterone. Vascular changes also occur in the muscular and skeletal systems which impact on how muscle and bone receive their nutrition.

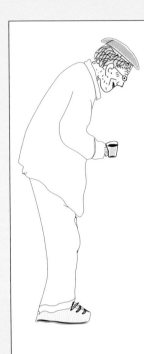

Respiratory system
- Loss of elastic recoil
- Reduced vital capacity
- Reduced inspiratory reserve volume
- Decrease in lung ventilation (increase in residual volume) leads to decreased oxygen diffusion into blood
- Reduced cough and ciliary action
- Increased chest wall rigidity

Cardiovascular system
- Reduced maximum heart rate
- Deposition of lipofuscin
- Reduced elasticity in arteries, build-up of fatty plaques
- Loss of sinoatrial node pacemaker cells
- Increased risk of heartbeat irregularities
- Reduced exercise tolerance

Musculoskeletal system
- Structural changes to the rib cage and spine, which impact on lung expansion and contraction
- Reduced bone density
- Reduced muscle mass due to reduced number and size of active muscle cells and decreased muscle strength
- Replacement of muscle cells with adipose tissue
- Loss of cartilage, loss of joint elasticity, cartilage calcification

FIGURE 13.1 Age-related changes and their impact on the respiratory, cardiovascular and musculoskeletal systems.

2. Climbing stairs requires a coordinated response from the cardiovascular, respiratory, renal, neuronal and endocrine systems. As David is 90 years of age, his coordination is not as effective as in someone who is middle aged, or in their early twenties. As he raises his legs to climb the stairs, his muscles will require increased energy and oxygen to manage this workload. Age-related changes in the healthy lung have not been shown to alter alveolar capacity in terms of affecting oxygen exchange across the alveolar wall; however, what is different is the age-related volume of air that is being inhaled and therefore available to be supplied to the circulation and that needs to reach the muscle. Hence, increased work by the musculoskeletal system, which also generates increased CO_2 and heat and needs an increase in oxygen supply, places an increased demand on the respiratory system to supply this oxygen need and effectively remove CO_2. In David's case, this manifests as shortness of breath, as his system tries to meet the demand.

3. The age-related changes in the lung affect the oxygenation of the skeletal muscles and the removal of muscle by-products of metabolic cell activity. However, the muscle stiffness experienced here is not due to the CO_2 or lactic acid accumulation arising as by-products that haven't been removed by respiratory system, but rather from decreased muscle elasticity and microscopic damage to the muscle.

BIBLIOGRAPHY

Bridge, N., & Tomkins, Z. (2020). Respiratory system. In Z. Tomkins (Ed.) *Applied anatomy and physiology – an interdisciplinary approach.* (1st ed.) (pp. 305–328). Chatswood, NSW: Elsevier.

Lee, M. (2020). Muscular system. In Z. Tomkins (Ed.) *Applied anatomy and physiology – an interdisciplinary approach.* (1st ed.) (pp. 103–112). Chatswood, NSW: Elsevier.

Lowery, E. M., Brubaker, A. L., Kuhlmann, E., & Kovacs, E. J. (2013). The aging lung. *Clinical Interventions in Aging,* 8, 1489–1496. doi: 10.2147/CIA.S51152.

Moore, S. (2020). The skeletal system. In Z. Tomkins (Ed.) *Applied anatomy and physiology – an interdisciplinary approach.* (1st ed.) (pp. 71–86). Chatswood, NSW: Elsevier.

Nelson, S., & Tomkins, Z. (2020). Cardiovascular system. In Z. Tomkins (Ed.) *Applied anatomy and physiology – an interdisciplinary approach.* (1st ed.) (pp. 227–248). Chatswood, NSW: Elsevier.

Roberts, S., Colombier, P., Sowman, A., Mennan, C., Rölfing, J. H., Guicheux, J., et al. (2016). Ageing in the musculoskeletal system. *Acta Orthopaedica,* 87(suppl 363), 15–25. doi: 10.1080/17453674.2016.1244750.

Strait, J. B., & Lakatta, E. G. (2012). Aging-associated cardiovascular changes and their relationship to heart failure. *Heart Failure Clinics,* 8(1), 143–164. doi: 10.1016/j.hfc.2011.08.011.

CASE 14
Teenagers' water endurance test

HISTORY

Jake and Edward are twins and are 15 years old. Jake is 1.76 metres tall, whereas Edward is 1.70 metres tall. They love living on the farm as each day they find a new challenge to conquer. Today, they have decided to submerge themselves into a 6-metre tank filled with water. To help them breathe under water, they found a 4-metre rigid tube of 1 cm diameter. Each boy boasted that they could stay under water for hours. Jake was first to go, while Edward was going to record how much time they may spend under the water. After 3 minutes, Jake emerged from the water feeling dizzy and gasping for air.

QUESTIONS

1. Under normal circumstances, what is the stimulus for breathing?

2. Considering gas exchange at the lung respiratory membrane and the anatomical dead space, suggest why Jake may be gasping for air.

3. Suggest why Jake became dizzy.

4. Had Jake not resurfaced when he did, what may have been the consequence?

ANSWERS: CASE 14
Teenagers' water endurance test

1. The most potent stimulus for breathing is increasing partial pressure of carbon dioxide (PCO_2) or an increasing concentration of CO_2. The peripheral chemoreceptors, located in the arterial aortic bodies and the carotid bodies (Figure 14.1), detect changes in the levels of O_2 and CO_2. Central chemoreceptors respond to changes in blood pH, which arise from changes in the levels of carbon dioxide in the blood. These receptors are located in the medulla oblongata in the vicinity of the medullar respiratory centre. Following these stimuli, the impulse generated by the peripheral chemoreceptors is conducted via nerves to the respiratory centres (medulla and pons). From there, efferent signals are sent to the diaphragm and the muscles of respiration to inhale and exhale air. Hypoxia, when the arterial O_2 falls below 60 mmHg, and acidaemia (H^+) will also stimulate the respiratory system to respond.

2. To understand why Jake would be gasping for air, it is necessary to review a few basic principles in the influence of CO_2 on lung ventilation. The anatomical dead space is the region of the respiratory system that conducts air to alveoli but where gas exchange does not occur. This includes the nose, trachea and bronchi. The physiological dead space is a sum of the anatomical dead space and the alveolar dead space, and it accounts for the volume of air that does not take part in gas exchange. This includes the bronchioles, alveolar ducts, alveolar sac and alveoli. In healthy humans, the anatomical dead space is estimated to be around 150 mL, whereas the alveolar dead space is deemed negligible. The respiratory membrane is a specialised structure (Figure 14.2) where air exchange occurs.

   Oxygen is inhaled from the atmosphere and is transported to the blood via diffusion across the respiratory membrane. Once in the blood, it is transported in two ways: (i) bound to haemoglobin molecules, where four molecules of oxygen bind to the haem porphyrin ring, and (ii) a very small amount is dissolved in plasma. The metabolic cell waste product, carbon dioxide (CO_2), is transported back to the lung in three ways: (i) as bicarbonate (HCO_3^-) dissolved in plasma (70%), (ii) as carbaminohaemoglobin, bound to haemoglobin (20%), and

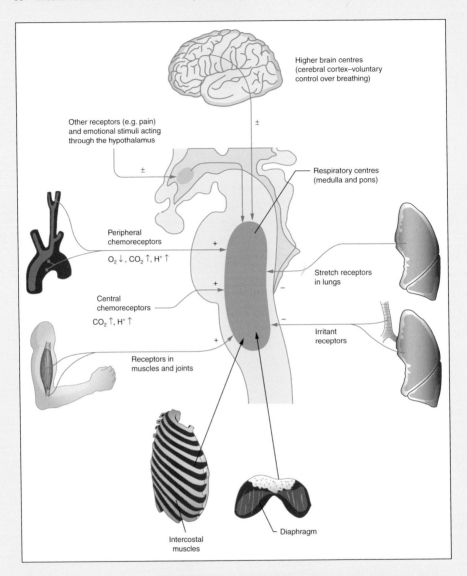

FIGURE 14.1 The stimulus to breathe comprises the following: afferent messages are sent to the respiratory centres in the brain from peripheral and central chemoreceptors, the respiratory system and peripheral receptors in muscles and joints. The respiratory centres then send signals to the intercostal muscles and the diaphragm to breathe in more air.

(iii) dissolved in plasma (10%) (Figure 14.3). Carbon dioxide is 20 times more soluble than O_2 so it quickly diffuses from tissue cells into the blood. Furthermore, reduced haemoglobin (oxygen free) can carry more CO_2 than does saturated haemoglobin. The affinity of haemoglobin for oxygen increases as more oxygen binds to the haem ring. This binding is also driven by the increased oxygen partial pressure (PO_2),

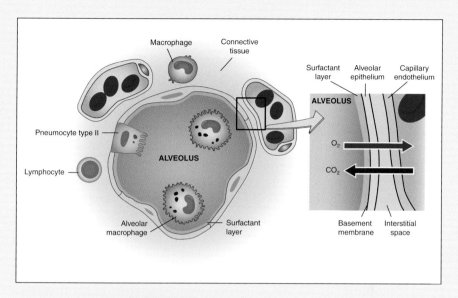

FIGURE 14.2 The respiratory membrane allows diffusion of oxygen from the air into the blood and diffusion of carbon dioxide into the air.

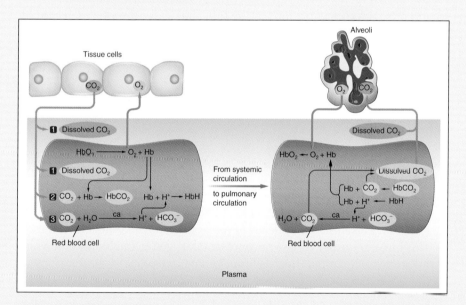

FIGURE 14.3 Transport of oxygen and carbon dioxide in the body. ca = carbonic anhydrase, Hb = haemoglobin.

which favours this interaction. The affinity of haemoglobin for O_2 diminishes as PO_2 decreases (from around 60 mmHg); therefore, oxygen is unloaded to peripheral tissue more readily. Clinically, the value of this information is that, at high PO_2 in the lungs, O_2 binds to haemoglobin whereas, in tissues where there is low PO_2, O_2 dissociates more readily from haemoglobin to enter tissue cells. This means that the porphyrin ring can undergo conformational change to free up spaces for CO_2 to bind more easily to haemoglobin, so it can form carbaminohaemoglobin and be carried back to the lung where it can be delivered to lung alveoli for removal from the body. This relationship is captured by the oxyhaemoglobin dissociation curve (see Figure 9.3).

As Jake breathed in through a long tube, this means that every time he exhaled some of that air would be trapped in the long tube as well as in the anatomical dead space (i.e. there was a greater reduction in alveolar ventilation). Hence, the concentration of oxygen would decrease and the concentration of carbon dioxide would increase. Every time Jake took a breath, he would breathe in a portion of the air that remained in the tube from his previous exhalation. A subsequent decrease in alveolar oxygen ventilation over time would lead to a build-up of CO_2 and nitrogen concentrations in the tube and in the alveoli. Such a build-up would result in hypercapnia, hypoxia and an increased respiratory rate (hyperpnoea). This last sign arises from CO_2 stimulation of the respiratory centres and is evident as an urgent need to breathe, resulting in hyperventilation (i.e. 'gasping for air') (Figure 14.4). The need to breathe is triggered primarily by the increased levels of CO_2 in the blood. Oxygen and plasma pH play lesser roles.

3. Jake became dizzy because the levels of CO_2 in his blood continued to increase, leading to hypercapnia, also known as hypercarbia. Dizziness arises from hyperventilation as Jake tries to remove excess CO_2 from his bloodstream. This leads to a rapid decrease in the partial pressure of CO_2 in the blood. As this event takes place, there is a concurrent development of respiratory alkalosis, which leads to vasoconstriction of brain blood vessels. This impairs the delivery of nutrients and oxygen to the brain cells, which collectively impair neuronal cell function and manifest as dizziness.

4. Hypercapnia, hypoxia and acidaemia combined with hyperventilation but without significant influence of pressure change would lead to loss of consciousness. Loss of consciousness is the result of complex central nervous system responses that involve the loss of adenosine triphosphate and associated loss of capacity to maintain the K^+/Na^+ pump and Ca^{2+} channels; in consequence, neurons that are deprived of oxygen start to reduce their activity, which is followed by loss of function if oxygen is not restored.

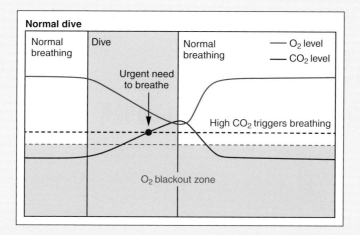

FIGURE 14.4 In a dive, the need to breathe is triggered primarily by increased levels of CO_2 in the blood. When the levels of CO_2 build up, this will stimulate the respiratory centres to send signals to intercostal muscles and the diaphragm to breathe in. Similarly, as the oxygen level falls below 60 mmHg, the resulting hypoxia will also stimulate the respiratory centres via the carotid body to increase the breathing. If the diver does not manage to breathe at the time of stimulation, loss of consciousness will occur.

BIBLIOGRAPHY

Bridge, N., & Tomkins, Z. (2020). Respiratory system. In Z. Tomkins (Ed.) *Applied anatomy and physiology – an interdisciplinary approach.* (1st ed.) (pp. 305–328). Chatswood, NSW: Elsevier.

Goodall, S., Twomey, R., & Amann, M. (2014). Acute and chronic hypoxia: implications for cerebral function and exercise tolerance. *Fatigue: Biomedicine, Health and Behavior,* 2(2), 73–92. doi: 10.1080/21641846.2014.909963.

Intagliata, S., Rizzo, A., & Gossman, W. G. (2020). Physiology, lung dead space. In *StatPearls* [Internet]. Treasure Island, FL: StatPearls Publishing. Available from: https://www.ncbi.nlm.nih.gov/books/NBK482501/.

Kettner, M., Ramsthaler, F., Juhnke, C., Bux, R., & Schmidt, P. (2013). A fatal case of CO(2) intoxication in a fermentation tank. *Journal of Forensic Science,* 58(2), 556–558.

Nelson, S., & Tomkins, Z. (2020). Cardiovascular system. In Z. Tomkins (Ed.) *Applied anatomy and physiology – an interdisciplinary approach.* (1st ed.) (pp. 227–248). Chatswood, NSW: Elsevier.

Permentier, K., Vercammen, S., Soetaert, S., & Schellemans, C. (2017). Carbon dioxide poisoning: a literature review of an often forgotten cause of intoxication in the emergency department. *International Journal of Emergency Medicine,* 10(1), 14.

Yap, K. (2020). Nervous system. In Z. Tomkins (Ed.) *Applied anatomy and physiology – an interdisciplinary approach.* (1st ed.) (pp. 113–134). Chatswood, NSW: Elsevier.

CASE 15
A woman with smoker's cough

HISTORY

Sophie is a 42-year-old mother of three. She does not smoke, but her partner, her mother and father all smoke. Sophie's partner smokes only outside of the house and, although she visits her parents often, she tries to avoid spending too much time indoors with them. Her parents have smoked for as long as she can remember. Sophie recently noticed that, when she gets up in the morning, she has a very productive cough and she finds that she must spit up large amounts of mucus that the cough brings. Some mornings, she wakes up with a crackling noise at the back of her throat. The cough lasts for several minutes and occasionally she also experiences it during the day. Concerned that she might have a chest infection, she visits her general practitioner (GP). After physical examination, the doctor suggests that she has a smoker's cough. The GP also proposes that Sophie takes a test that examines her lung's function to assess the lung volume and lung capacity.

QUESTIONS

1. Although Sophie is not a smoker, suggest why she might have developed a smoker's cough. What is the purpose of the cough?

2. Explain why she would be producing an increased volume of mucus.

3. Consider what impact an increased presence of mucus arising from chronic exposure to cigarette smoke may have on the gas exchange function of the lung.

4. Explain the purpose of lung function tests and suggest why these would be requested by the GP.

ANSWERS: CASE 15
A woman with smoker's cough

1. Sophie has been exposed to toxic particles present in the cigarette smoke through passive inhalation. This is often referred to as passive smoking. The particles irritate the respiratory tract by causing it injury. In response to the injury, the respiratory system responds by activating the inflammatory response, which includes cough. Cough is a natural reflex aimed at moving offending irritant towards the pharynx so that it is then either swallowed or expectorated. The cough is initiated when the nerve fibres in the lung detect the presence of the irritant via chemoreceptors, and then convey the message via afferent impulses carried by the vagus nerve to the cough reflex centre in the medulla oblongata (central nervous system) (Figure 15.1). The efferent impulses generated there travel via parasympathetic and motor nerves to the diaphragm, intercostal muscles and lung to cause increased contraction of the diaphragmatic, abdominal and intercostal muscles to help produce a cough. It is also suggested that the cough reflex centre is neuronally connected to the respiratory centres in the brain and that this connection enables control of the breathing pattern needed to produce a cough. This collaboration between the cough reflex centre and the respiratory centres is thought to be responsible for generating the combination of rapid inspiration, increase of intrapulmonary pressure and expiration against a closed glottis that produces sufficient force for a high-velocity, upward-travelling expiration of gas and mucus once the glottis is opened.

   The injury can span from the alveoli to bronchi. The effect that passive smoking has on an individual would vary, depending on the dose and frequency of exposure. People who are more frequently exposed to higher concentrations of cigarette smoke are likely to experience more severe forms of lung injury.

2. The healthy epithelial cells lining the lower respiratory tract produce secretions that have a protective function as they clear foreign particles. This is possible because the motile cilia which

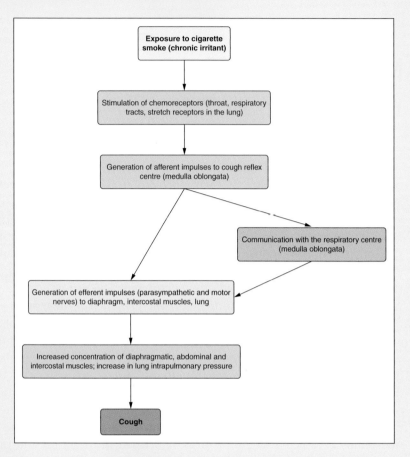

FIGURE 15.1 Simplified schematic representation of cough mechanisms in response to cigarette smoke.

line the epithelial tract rhythmically sweep the secretion upwards towards the pharynx. These secretions are swallowed. Note that the secretions contain small amounts of mucus, which is produced by the goblet cells, also found in the respiratory epithelium. In the presence of increased concentration of irritating particles found in cigarette smoke, the secretions become enriched in mucus (Figure 15.2). The increased mucus production increases the viscosity of the lung secretions, making them stickier (see Figure 15.3). Mucus also contains various chemicals, antibodies and immune cells whose function is to eliminate the offending particle. In chronic exposure to cigarette smoke, the cilia lining the epithelium are increasingly

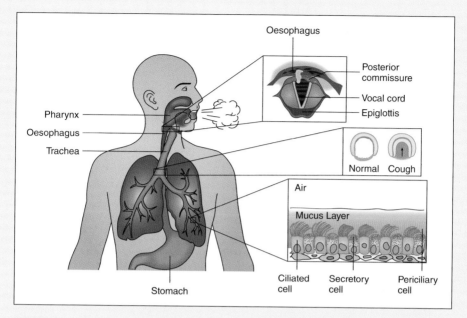

FIGURE 15.2 Mucus is secreted by the goblet cells of the bronchial epithelium (bottom right). In healthy lungs the resulting mucus is moved by the cilia towards the pharynx and would be swallowed into the oesophagus. Increased production of mucus and impaired ciliary movement arising from chronic exposure to smoke activate the cough reflex to propel the mucus forcefully towards the pharynx where it is either swallowed or expectorated.
Source: Visual Art ©2018. The University of Texas, MD Anderson Cancer Center.

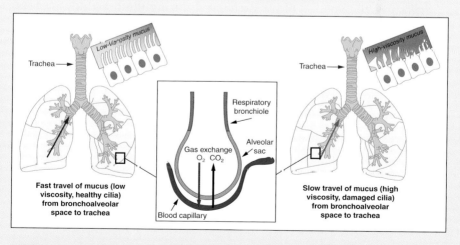

FIGURE 15.3 Increased mucus secretions that have an impaired clearance from the lungs will impair the capacity of oxygen to diffuse across the respiratory membrane.

damaged and their capacity to continually sweep the mucus towards the pharynx would also be impaired. Hence, failure to remove the mucus leads to mucus accumulation. As accumulation of the mucus would lead to impaired air exchange and increasing irritation of the lung chemoreceptors, this would cause Sophie to cough.

3. The gas exchange occurs at the alveolar level (Figure 15.3). There oxygen, which was delivered into the lung during the process of inspiration, diffuses across the alveolar respiratory membrane epithelium via the endothelial cells into the blood, where they bind to haemoglobin located in the red blood cells. The oxygenated blood is then transported by the branches of pulmonary vein to the heart for systemic distribution. Deoxygenated blood is transported by the branches of pulmonary artery to the lung capillaries, which enable CO_2 to diffuse from blood into alveoli for a release into the atmosphere during the expiration process. When there is a build-up of mucus in the alveolar structures then the passage of oxygen into the blood is impaired, as the distance that oxygen needs to travel to diffuse into the blood has increased. Furthermore, as the mucus occupies a volume of space in the lung alveoli, there is a reduction in airway diameter so less oxygen can be delivered into the alveoli. When less oxygen diffuses into the blood, there is less oxygen available for tissues to use for chemical processes. Compensatory mechanisms are then activated, one of which is to breathe more deeply and more frequently to increase the oxygen uptake.

4. The purpose of the lung function tests is to measure lung volume, lung capacity, rate of air flow and gas exchange capacity. A spirometer, which measures the volume of air exchanged during the breathing process, is used to determine the tidal volume (the volume of air exhaled after inspiration), the expiratory reserve volume (the greatest volume of air exhaled forcibly after the tidal volume of air is exhaled), the inspiratory reserve volume (the volume of air inspired forcibly above normal inspiration) and the residual volume (the volume of air that cannot be forcibly expired) (Figure 15.4A, B).

   The results help to evaluate the lung function and aid the clinician to diagnose the respiratory condition correctly and choose the best evidence-based treatment. The tests also allow the clinician to determine the baseline at the time of patient presentation and evaluate the progress of the condition during follow-up.

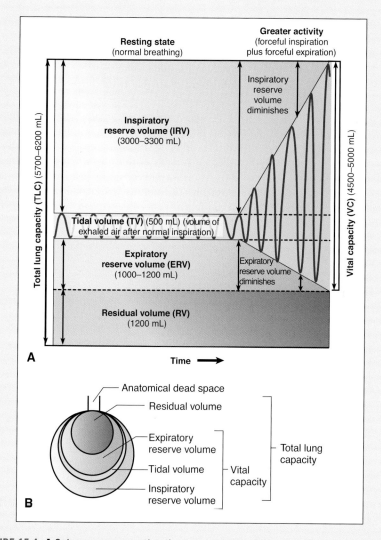

FIGURE 15.4 A Spirogram representing the measurement of the volume of gas that the healthy lungs may inhale and exhale over a specific period of time. **B** Pulmonary volumes (at rest) demonstrated as relative proportions of an inhaled balloon.

BIBLIOGRAPHY

Abdelkader, A., & Barbagallo, M. S. (2020). Immune system. In Z. Tomkins (Ed.) *Applied anatomy and physiology – an interdisciplinary approach.* (1st ed.) (pp. 265–278). Chatswood, NSW: Elsevier.

Bridge, N., & Tomkins, Z. (2020). Respiratory system. In Z. Tomkins (Ed.) *Applied anatomy and physiology – an interdisciplinary approach.* (1st ed.) (pp. 305–328). Chatswood, NSW: Elsevier.

Dickey, B. F. (2018). What it takes for a cough to expel mucus from the airway. *Proceedings of the National Academy of Sciences of the United States of America*, 115(49), 12340–12342. doi: 10.1073/pnas.1817484115.

Lofrese, J. J., & Lappin, S. L. (2020). Physiology, residual volume. In *StatPearls* [Internet]. Treasure Island, FL: StatPearls Publishing. Available from: https://www.ncbi.nlm.nih.gov/books/NBK493170/.

Office on Smoking and Health (US). (2006). *The health consequences of involuntary exposure to tobacco smoke: a report of the Surgeon General.* (Chapter 9, Respiratory effects in adults from exposure to secondhand smoke). Atlanta, GA: Centers for Disease Control and Prevention (US). Available from: https://www.ncbi.nlm.nih.gov/books/NBK44316/.

Tomkins, Z. (2020). Acute inflammation. In Z. Tomkins (Ed.) *Applied anatomy and physiology – an interdisciplinary approach.* (1st ed.) (pp. 279–304). Chatswood, NSW: Elsevier.

CASE 16
A truck driver with anal fissure

HISTORY

Sarah is a 56-year-old truck driver who drives long distances across Australia. Today she was driving from Melbourne to Adelaide, where she lives. Sarah is a busy truck driver and often eats a diet that does not contain enough fibre and valuable nutrition. For the past 4 days, Sarah hasn't opened her bowels, which is not normal for her. Today, she felt bloated and felt a constant need to try to open her bowels. Despite going to the toilet and straining a lot, she managed, after being on the toilet for 15 minutes, to pass a very hard piece of stool. During defecation, Sarah felt a sharp pain in her anus. When she wiped her bottom, bright red blood stained the toilet paper. Back in her truck, Sarah found it extremely painful to sit down and drive. Experiencing a lot of pain and discomfort for the next 6 hours, she took painkillers to get through to Adelaide. When she felt that she needed to open her bowels again, she again passed a hard piece of stool and the pain returned. She called her family clinic to make an appointment with the doctor. At the clinic, Sarah explained to the doctor what had happened and she expressed strong concern about needing to pass stools again and the degree of pain she anticipated she might experience. On rectal examination the doctor saw a posterior anal fissure: a tear in the anoderm. The doctor explained that, although treatments are available, the fundamental change that needs to be made is for Sarah to change her diet by increasing her dietary fibre and water intake.

QUESTIONS

1. Explain why an anal fissure might have occurred.

2. Explain why Sarah felt so much pain at the site of the fissure.

3. Considering that the anus is a site of expulsion of faeces, what tissue repair reactions would you expect at this site, and how do inflammation and immune reactions impact on the defecation function in Sarah's case?

4. Discuss why fibre and water intake is important for keeping the stools soft and the bowel motion regular.

ANSWERS: CASE 16
A truck driver with anal fissure

1. Constipation and passage of hard stools are associated with the development of an anal fissure (a tear in the anus) (Figure 16.1). It is proposed that this occurs as a result of overstretching of the anoderm, a squamous epithelial lining of the anus. Most anal fissures are located in

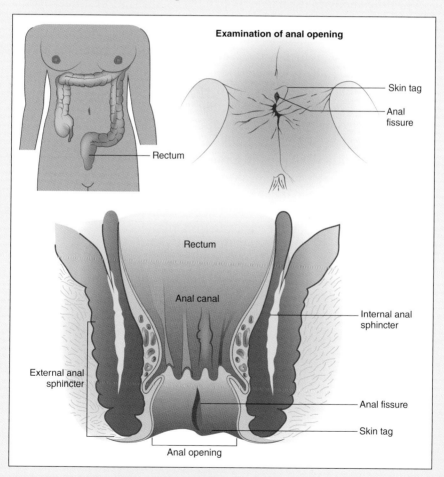

FIGURE 16.1 Schematic representation of an anal fissure.

the midline and are predominantly posterior; however, the reason for this pattern is unknown.

2. The pain experienced is due to the tearing of the anoderm and the stimulation of local nociceptors, and possibly reopening of the tear each time the bowel motion occurs. The pain contributes to the causes of spasm of the anal sphincter muscle. This is a protective mechanism aimed at preventing further stretching and tearing of the anus. However, these spasms also cause vasoconstriction, which leads to ischaemic episodes in the anorectal muscle. As the spasm occurs every time a bowel motion occurs, the ischaemia is exacerbated, which impairs the healing rate of the anal fissure. This recurrent event leads to chronic anal spasms and persistent pain.

3. A healthy anoderm is a barrier to pathogens, such as intestinal bacteria. Note that, although intestinal bacteria have commensal value in human health while in the intestine, they can have a pathogenic effect if they enter the human body elsewhere. An anal fissure is a wound in the anoderm. To close the wound, the local region will activate acute inflammation, which is characterised by localised increase in blood flow, heat, swelling, pain and, in Sarah's case, a degree of impaired function (passing stools was a painful experience). Wound repair also includes activation of local innate and adaptive immune responses, including synthesis of pro-inflammatory cytokines. Increased vascular permeability that leads to localised tissue oedema, evident as swelling of the tissue, would impact on the function of the anal sphincter muscle. Nociceptors in the local area become sensitised further, owing to localised prostaglandin release arising from local tissue destruction. As stools are passed through the anus, the injured area would be continuously exposed to intestinal bacteria. Immune cells present in the anoderm would persistently engage in managing any of the intestinal bacteria that may enter the wound, so preventing infection. If the anal tear were not healing, these reactions would continue to contribute to cycles of spasms and pain, further complicating the healing process.

4. As food is passed through the digestive system, it will be subjected to chemical digestion. This will facilitate food breakdown towards absorbable units such as proteins, fats and carbohydrates. When stools are formed, they are composed of materials that have not been digested. Constipation occurs when the contents in the distal rectum move at a reduced rate compared with what would be normal for the person. This means that the contents spend more time in the rectum, enabling

more water to be absorbed from the faecal matter and so leading to the production of hardened stool. Dietary fibre, both soluble and insoluble, increases the weight and bulk of stools and softens the stools. It does this by absorbing the water in the intestine. This results in easier defecation. This is the reason why the doctor advised Sarah to drink more water. Failure to do so may cause the fibre to itself become a constipating agent.

BIBLIOGRAPHY

Beaty, J. S., & Shashidharan, M. (2016). Anal fissure. *Clinics in Colon and Rectal Surgery*, 29(1), 30–37. doi: 10.1055/s-0035-1570390.

Higuero, T. (2016). Update on the management of anal fissure. *Journal of Visceral Surgery*, 152(2), S37–S43.

Kapp, S., & Tomkins, Z. (2020). Integumentary system. In Z. Tomkins (Ed.) *Applied anatomy and physiology – an interdisciplinary approach.* (1st ed.) (pp. 53–70). Chatswood, NSW: Elsevier.

Lang, E. (2020). Nutrition and metabolism. In Z. Tomkins (Ed.) *Applied anatomy and physiology – an interdisciplinary approach.* (1st ed.) (pp. 349–360). Chatswood, NSW: Elsevier.

On, W. H., Lim, Y. J., & Yap, K. (2020). Gastrointestinal system. In Z. Tomkins (Ed.) *Applied anatomy and physiology – an interdisciplinary approach.* (1st ed.) (pp. 329–348). Chatswood, NSW: Elsevier.

Sugerman, D. T. (2014). Anal fissure. *Journal of the American Medical Association*, 311(11), 1171. doi: 10.1001/jama.2014.214.

Tomkins, Z. (2020). Acute inflammation. In Z. Tomkins (Ed.) *Applied anatomy and physiology – an interdisciplinary approach.* (1st ed.) (pp. 279–304). Chatswood, NSW: Elsevier.

Yang, J., Wang, H. P., Zhou, L., & Xu, C. F. (2012). Effect of dietary fiber on constipation: a meta analysis. *World Journal of Gastroenterology*, 18(48), 7378–7383. doi:10.3748/wjg.v18.i48.7378.

Yap, K. (2020). Nervous system. In Z. Tomkins (Ed.) *Applied anatomy and physiology – an interdisciplinary approach.* (1st ed.) (pp. 113–134). Chatswood, NSW: Elsevier.

CASE 17
Food poisoning

HISTORY

Monica is a postdoctoral scientist. After spending 12 hours in the lab, she and her colleagues went out to a local restaurant to have dinner. Monica ordered char-grilled eggplant covered in Parmesan cheese and barbequed chicken. She drank water with her dinner. After dinner, Monica went home to bed and fell asleep quickly. Around 4 o'clock in the morning, she woke up feeling unwell. As she sat up, she felt a strong wave of nausea and rushed to the bathroom, where she started to retch but did not vomit. She returned to her bedroom, but the nausea persisted. She tried to lie down to make herself more comfortable. However, as she did so, she felt the contents of her stomach in her mouth and she managed to reach the bathroom, where she vomited. For the next 4 hours she continued to retch and vomit, and in the morning she also developed diarrhoea. Monica phoned the local clinic, where she was seen by a general practitioner.

QUESTIONS

1. What might have caused the nausea and what are the physiological mechanisms likely to explain this in Monica's case?

2. What is the physiological mechanism of emesis (the act of vomiting)?

3. Describe the difference between retching and vomiting.

4. Discuss the role of emesis in maintaining immunological barriers and preventing infections.

5. Discuss the consequence of prolonged nausea and vomiting on other body systems.

6. Explain why diarrhoea has occurred in this case.

ANSWERS: CASE 17
Food poisoning

1. Nausea is the feeling of wanting to vomit, but not the act of vomiting. Although there are many causes of nausea, in Monica's case it is likely to be due to toxins secreted by bacteria that were ingested in contaminated food and the bacteria itself as they attempt to infect the gastric mucosa.

2. In Monica's case, the toxins secreted by the bacteria in the stomach and intestinal lumen will stimulate enterochromaffin cells in the stomach and gut mucosa (Figure 17.1). These will release inflammatory mediators such as 5-hydroxytryptophan (5-HT), commonly known as serotonin. Some of the toxins may also directly enter the bloodstream and travel to the brain. Serotonin will depolarise sensory afferent neurons in the gut mucosa via $5-HT_3$ receptors. This will lead to formation of an action potential in afferent vagal nerves and its conduction to the brain stem, where the chemoreceptor trigger zone is located. The chemoreceptor trigger zone receptors are located in the area postrema (found in the floor of the fourth ventricle within the brain) and, as it is located outside the blood–brain barrier, this area is directly exposed to noxious stimuli arriving via the bloodstream and cerebrospinal fluid. Afferent signals will also be relayed via the brain stem to the nucleus of the solitary tract (nucleus tractus solidarius). In addition to toxins, other stimuli can be due to local inflammation, where localised oedema and swelling stimulate mechanoreceptors in the gastrointestinal tract and generate an action potential that is then conducted via the vagus nerve to the central nervous system to elicit a response.

   The afferent signals are processed by the vomiting centre, which is located in the reticular formation of the medulla oblongata, close to the respiratory centre. The efferent signals are sent to the diaphragm, abdominal muscles, oesophagus and visceral nerves of the stomach to induce the feeling of nausea (arising from reduced gastric motility) and vomiting, as well as to activate the autonomic nervous system via the vagal nerve. This is followed by a decrease in peristaltic activity within the small intestine, regurgitation of the intestinal content into the stomach, contraction of the diaphragm and the abdominal muscles and lowering of the diaphragm against a closed glottis. This forces the stomach content into the oesophagus and out of the mouth.

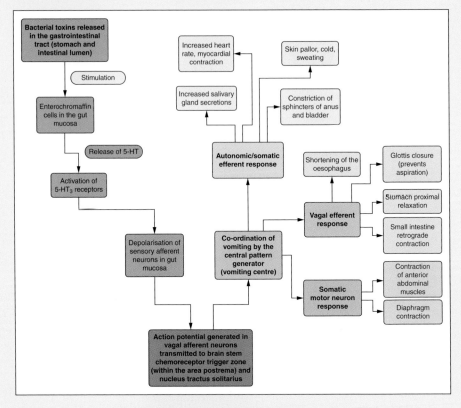

FIGURE 17.1 Bacterial food poisoning-associated activation of vomiting.

3. Retching and vomiting are both involuntary processes. Both involve the diaphragm and abdominal muscles with the glottis closed. However, during retching no gastric contents are expulsed, whereas during vomiting the contents are expelled. Retching involves deep inspiration against a closed glottis. Speech is not possible during retching. Note that retching can precede vomiting; however, it can also occur on its own – for example, when caused by a bad smell or severe stress.

4. Vomiting provides a means of removing gastrointestinal contents that are irritating the digestive system. This action is thought to comprise part of the innate defence mechanism, as it removes bacteria and their products thus reducing the chance of extensive irritation and wounding to the cells lining the digestive tract, from the pharynx, oesophagus and stomach to the upper part of the small intestine.

5. During vomiting, respiration is inhibited. The epiglottis and soft palate close off the trachea and nasopharynx to prevent the vomitus from

being inhaled (aspirated). If gastric acid or food enters the airway, it will cause damage indicative of aspiration pneumonia. Vomiting can induce loss of fluid (dehydration), electrolyte imbalance and disturbance of the acid–base balance in the body. The electrolyte imbalance comes from loss of acid (H^+ ions) and chloride (Cl^-) as the kidneys compensate for the loss of acid through secreting potassium ions (K^+) into the urine. Severe vomiting can also lead to vomiting of bile.

6. Similarly to the induction of vomiting, bacterial toxins released in the gastrointestinal tract act on the intestinal cells. Here the toxins cause mucosal irritation and increased mucous secretion. This can be accompanied by excessive secretion of electrolytes and fluid. This type of large-volume diarrhoea, caused by excessive mucosal secretions enriched with chloride or bicarbonate and sodium, is known as secretory diarrhoea. The role of the increased volume of fluid is to wash away the infectious particles from the gut. Combined with increased gastrointestinal motility, the aim is to move the infected contents quickly towards the anus for excretion. This does not allow the reabsorption of the water in the large intestine, and so diarrhoea ensues.

BIBLIOGRAPHY

Abdelkader, A., & Barbagallo, M. S. (2020). Immune system. In Z. Tomkins (Ed.) *Applied anatomy and physiology – an interdisciplinary approach.* (1st ed.) (pp. 265–278). Chatswood, NSW: Elsevier.

Chow, C. M., Leung, A. K., & Hon, K. L. (2010). Acute gastroenteritis: from guidelines to real life. *Clinical and Experimental Gastroenterology,* 3, 97–112. doi: 10.2147/ceg. s6554.

On, W. H., Lim, Y. J., & Yap, K. (2020). Gastrointestinal system. In Z. Tomkins (Ed.) *Applied anatomy and physiology – an interdisciplinary approach.* (1st ed.) (pp. 329–348). Chatswood, NSW: Elsevier.

Singh, P., Yoon, S. S., & Kuo, B. (2016). Nausea: a review of pathophysiology and therapeutics. *Therapeutic Advances in Gastroenterology,* 9(1), 98–112. doi: 10.1177/1756283X15618131.

Sivakumar, S., & Prabhu, A. (2020). Physiology, gag reflex. In *StatPearls* [Internet]. Treasure Island, FL: StatPearls PublishingAvailable from: https://www.ncbi.nlm. nih.gov/books/NBK554502/.

Tomkins, Z. (2020). Acute inflammation. In Z. Tomkins (Ed.) *Applied anatomy and physiology – an interdisciplinary approach.* (1st ed.) (pp. 279 304). Chatswood, NSW: Elsevier.

CASE 18
An elderly lady with dehydration

HISTORY

Alma is a healthy 85-year-old woman with no previous significant medical history. She has lived on a farm all her life and actively participated in the work on the farm. As she became older, her passions were directed to her rose garden. Today, the weather was expected to reach 45°C, and Alma was worried about her roses surviving the heat. Although she went into the garden at around 8 o'clock in the morning and took small breaks to rest, Alma forgot about the time. Her granddaughter, Ella, brought her a cup of tea in the morning and then again at lunchtime, urging her grandmother to come inside the house where it was cooler. By that point, Alma had already been in her garden for 5 hours, which she spent mostly sitting on a gardening pillow, and was covered in sweat. Alma agreed to come inside as she had completed the work she wanted to do, and she admitted to feeling quite dehydrated. Ella helped her to her feet, but when Alma stood up she felt dizzy. Ella helped her into the house, where Ella helped Alma to sit down and then called for help, worried that her grandmother may become unwell.

QUESTIONS

1. What is the role of perspiration during a hot day?

2. Explain why Alma might have felt dehydrated and dizzy.

3. Explain how Alma's renal system would respond to the loss of water through perspiration and low intake of water in this situation.

4. Why was it important for Alma to sit down when feeling dizzy?

ANSWERS: CASE 18
An elderly lady with dehydration

1. The role of perspiration or sweating is to release body heat. The homeostatic temperature range for a healthy human is 36.5–37.5°C (Figure 18.1). An increase in body heat, arising from exposure to environmental heat in Alma's case, will increase blood temperature. It will also stimulate nerve receptors in the skin, which will send signals to the hypothalamus. Simultaneously, as the blood passes through the hypothalamus, it will also be sensed by the hypothalamic centre. In turn, the hypothalamus will activate the heat loss mechanisms. These mechanisms involve arteriolar and capillary (effectors) vasodilation near the skin surface to facilitate heat release from the blood into the environment. This causes erector muscles (effectors) in the skin to relax so that the skin hair can lie flat on the skin, hence trapping less hot air. Arterioles supplying the sweat glands (effectors) also dilate and bring a higher volume of blood to the glands so that the sweat glands can lose heat in the form of increased sweat excretion. The sweat excretion leads to heat loss through evaporation from the skin surface.

2. Alma would have lost a volume of water through perspiration as well as her low intake of fluids on the hot day. This would result in lower intravascular volume available for circulation and so her blood pressure would decrease (Figure 18.2). When Alma stood up suddenly, she experienced orthostatic hypotension, also known as postural hypotension. Several events would have led to this experience. As she was sweating, her blood vessels would be dilated, meaning that a volume of blood was redistributed away from the central vasculature. Because she was kneeling, some of the blood would pool in her venous circulation, which means that there would be a decrease in cardiac output. This would activate the baroreceptors to respond. In addition, gravity would influence her vestibular system: the blood would need to travel up to the brain against gravity, which would result in reduced perfusion of the brain vasculature. Hence, her brain would temporarily be receiving a reduced blood supply, which would activate the cerebral autoregulation centre to re-establish the blood pressure needed to maintain blood perfusion to the brain. It also means that the brain cells may temporarily receive a decreased volume of oxygen.

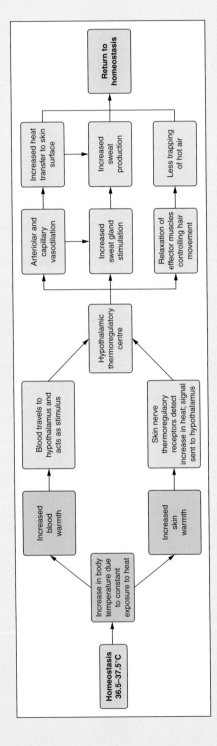

FIGURE 18.1 Mechanisms of heat release through perspiration.

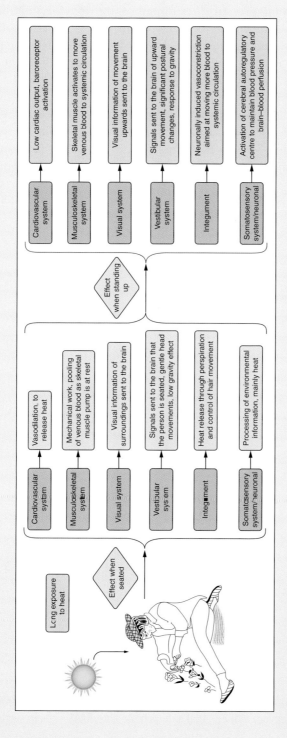

FIGURE 18.2 Complex interactions occur among multiple body systems to help Alma adjust from her position of sitting down to the position of standing upright. The culmination of the response is adequate vascular perfusion of the brain – the master regulator of all physiological functions.

3. A drop in blood pressure accompanies the loss of fluid from the internal body environment. This event causes the hypothalamus to release antidiuretic hormone (ADH) from the posterior pituitary gland (Figure 18.3). ADH increases water reabsorption by the kidneys as it increases water permeability of the distal tubules and collecting ducts. The drop in blood pressure is also detected by each nephron's juxtaglomerular apparatus, which responds by secreting renin. Renin triggers the formation of angiotensin I from its precursor angiotensinogen, which is formed by the liver. Angiotensin I is converted to angiotensin II by angiotensin converting enzyme (ACE),

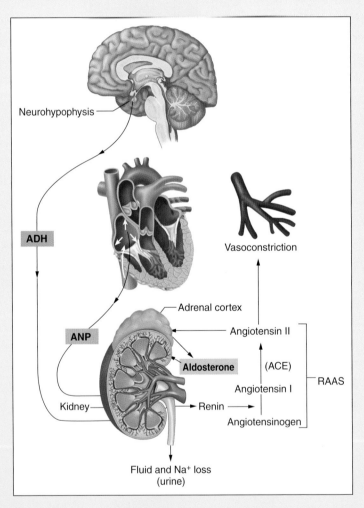

FIGURE 18.3 The renal response to dehydration. ACE = angiotensin converting enzyme, ADH = antidiuretic hormone, ANP = atrial natriuretic peptide, RAAS = renin–angiotensin–aldosterone system.

which is mostly found in the lung capillaries. Angiotensin II causes vasoconstriction and acts on the adrenal cortex to stimulate the release of aldosterone. Aldosterone then slowly boosts water reabsorption by the kidneys by increasing reabsorption of sodium ions (Na^+). Because angiotensin II also stimulates the secretion of ADH, it serves as an additional link between the ADH and aldosterone mechanisms. The drop in intravascular blood volume also inhibits atrial natriuretic peptide (ANP), which would otherwise act to promote loss of water and sodium by the kidneys.

4. It is important that Alma allows her body to adjust to the postural change and for it to respond to the decreased vascular volume arising from dehydration. Sitting down helps this process; it would also minimise her risk of falls if she were to develop syncope (temporary loss of consciousness due to decreased blood supply to the brain) and thus prevent further injury such as bone fractures.

BIBLIOGRAPHY

Dmitrieva, N. I., & Burg, M. B. (2011). Increased insensible water loss contributes to aging related dehydration. *PloS One*, 6(5), e20691.

Goswami, N., Blaber, A. P., Hinghofer-Szalkay, H., & Montani, J. P. (2017). Orthostatic intolerance in older persons: etiology and countermeasures. *Frontiers in Physiology*, 8, 803.

Hooper, L., Bunn, D., Jimoh, F. O., & Fairweather-Tait, S. J. (2014). Water-loss dehydration and aging. *Mechanisms of Ageing and Development*, 136–137, 50–58.

Kapp, S., & Tomkins, Z. (2020). Integumentary system. In Z. Tomkins (Ed.) *Applied anatomy and physiology – an interdisciplinary approach.* (1st ed.) (pp. 53–70). Chatswood, NSW: Elsevier.

Montayre, J., Macdiarmid, R., McDonald, E. M., & Saravanakumar, P. (2020). Urinary system. In Z. Tomkins (Ed.) *Applied anatomy and physiology – an interdisciplinary approach.* (1st ed.) (pp. 361–382). Chatswood, NSW: Elsevier.

Nelson, S., & Tomkins, Z. (2020). Cardiovascular system. In Z. Tomkins (Ed.) *Applied anatomy and physiology – an interdisciplinary approach.* (1st ed.) (pp. 227–248). Chatswood, NSW: Elsevier.

Yap, K. (2020). Nervous system. In Z. Tomkins (Ed.) *Applied anatomy and physiology – an interdisciplinary approach.* (1st ed.) (pp. 113–134). Chatswood, NSW: Elsevier.

CASE 19
Ectopic pregnancy

HISTORY

Amber is a 33-year-old executive who presented to the emergency department after experiencing persistent severe sharp, intermittent abdominal pain in the left lower quadrant for the past 2 hours. She also had pain in her left shoulder. On assessment, the attending doctor did a pelvic exam, and then asked Amber if she might be pregnant. Amber stated that, to her knowledge, she was not, but that she and her partner were trying to get pregnant. Her last period was 6 weeks ago. The doctor ordered an urgent ultrasound and requested a blood test for human chorionic gonadotropin (hCG) to eliminate the possibility that Amber might be pregnant. Amber has no other significant medical history.

QUESTIONS

1. In a normal pregnancy, describe the anatomical locations where the ovum is most likely to be fertilised and the journey to the implantation site in the uterus.

2. Discuss what an ectopic pregnancy is and how it may lead to severe abdominal pain and shoulder pain as experienced by Amber.

3. Why is ectopic pregnancy a medical emergency?

4. Would you expect that, in the early stages, the ectopic pregnancy has the same symptoms as normal pregnancy? Provide a rationale for your answer.

5. Discuss the source of hCG and its diagnostic value in ectopic pregnancy.

ANSWERS: CASE 19
Ectopic pregnancy

1. In general, following ovulation, where the oocyte is expulsed from the mature ovarian follicle into the abdominopelvic cavity, the oocyte enters the fallopian (uterine) tubes (Figure 19.1). There, it may unite with one of many millions of sperm, which signals that the fertilisation has

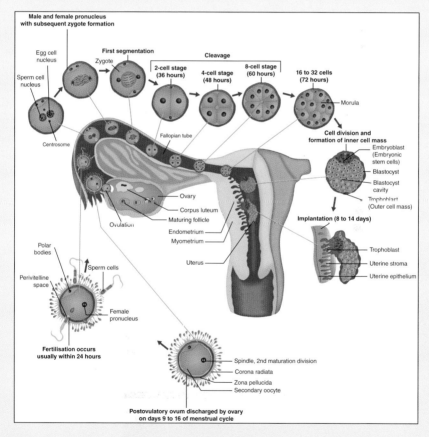

FIGURE 19.1 Fertilisation of the ovum and implantation into the uterine wall. Note that, following fertilisation in a fallopian tube, the fertilised ovum (zygote) goes through a rapid cell division to form a morula and then transforms into a blastocyst. Once implantation occurs, the embryo will continue to develop.

occurred. Fertilisation leads to the formation of the zygote. The zygote then undergoes an embryogenesis process, which is characterised by rapid cellular divisions and cleavages over approximately a 3-day period to develop into a morula. The morula undergoes transformational change as it continues to travel towards the uterus. This transport is dependent on complex interactions between the epithelium lining the fallopian tube, the fluid content in the fallopian tube and any contents in the tube. The interaction between these anatomical components are evident as tubal peristalsis, epithelial ciliary motion and tubal fluid flow, which combine to generate a mechanical force that will move the morula towards the uterine cavity. Over the next few days the morula develops into a hollow ball-like mass of cells, termed a blastocyst. The blastocyst will then implant, approximately 8 days after fertilisation, into the uterine endometrial wall.

2. Ectopic pregnancy is a term used to describe the implantation of the fertilised egg in anatomical sites other than the uterine cavity (Figure 19.2). As the embryo grows, it stretches the fallopian tube. Fallopian tubes contain afferent pain fibres, which travel along the same pathway as sympathetic efferent innervation. Minor parasympathetic innervation is also present. Hence, as the implanted embryo increases in size and it stretches the surrounding fallopian tube, it will cause localised tissue damage and release prostaglandins that will activate the visceral nociceptors. Similarly, mechanical stretch will also stimulate nociceptors. Bleeding that may leak into the abdominal cavity may irritate the diaphragm and lead to referred shoulder pain.

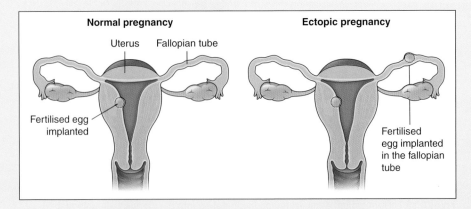

FIGURE 19.2 Implantation in normal pregnancy and in ectopic pregnancy.
©Mayo Clinic.

3. The implantation of the fertilised egg in anatomical locations that cannot stretch and accommodate the growing fetus means that the tissue will overstretch and eventually rupture. Such rupture can lead to significant haemorrhage, which can lead to maternal death.

4. Yes, as in the early stages of pregnancy the process of fertilisation and embryonic cell division would be the same until the fallopian tube could no longer support the implanted embryo. Hormonal changes in those early stages of pregnancy would be the same as in a normal pregnancy. This means that the pregnancy test would be positive in both cases; a missed period would be expected in both presentations, as would breast tenderness and nausea. Note, however, that each person responds differently to pregnancy hormones, so nausea may not be present in all cases.

5. Human chorionic gonadotropin (hCG) is synthesised and released by the embryonic trophoblast cells, which help to maintain the viability of corpus luteum. The corpus luteum is responsible for the production of oestrogen and progesterone hormones, which are needed to maintain uterine function in supporting the early stages of pregnancy. Oestrogen stimulates the growth of myometrium and prepares the mammary glands for lactation. Progesterone will suppress uterine contraction and help to prepare the mammary glands for lactation. In normal pregnancy, it would be expected that the serum concentrations of hCG would increase during early pregnancy, and this is often used to estimate the embryonic gestational stage (Figure 19.3). In Amber's case, hCG would be used to confirm the pregnancy. Note that this test cannot be used to confirm an ectopic pregnancy. For that purpose, a high-resolution transvaginal ultrasound (where safe) and/or transabdominal ultrasound will be used.

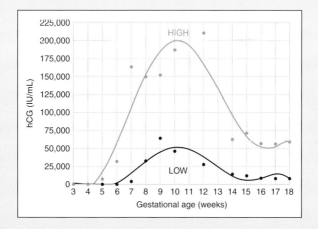

FIGURE 19.3 Reference ranges for human chorionic gonadotropin (hCG) during the first 18 weeks of pregnancy.
©2019 Focus Information Technology.

BIBLIOGRAPHY

Barnhart, K. T., Guo, W., Cary, M. S., Morse, C. B., Chung, K., Takacs, P., et al. (2016). Differences in serum human chorionic gonadotropin rise in early pregnancy by race and value at presentation. *Obstetrics and Gynecology*, 128(3), 504–511. doi: 10.1097/AOG.0000000000001568.

BMJ Best Practice. (2020). Ectopic pregnancy. Available from: https://bestpractice.bmj. com/topics/en-gb/174.

Byrne, J. H. (Ed.) (2020) *Neuroscience online: an electronic textbook for the neurosciences.* Houston, TX: TMC Department of Neurobiology and Anatomy. Available from: http://nba.uth.tmc.edu/neuroscience/.

Carr, B. (2020). Pregnancy and lactation. In Z. Tomkins (Ed.) *Applied anatomy and physiology – an interdisciplinary approach.* (1st ed.) (pp. 399–414). Chatswood, NSW: Elsevier.

Han, J., & Sadiq, N. M. (2020). Anatomy, abdomen and pelvis, fallopian tube. In *StatPearls* [Internet]. Treasure Island, FL: StatPearls Publishing. Available from: https://www.ncbi.nlm.nih.gov/books/NBK547660/.

Korevaar, T. I., Steegers, E. A., de Rijke, Y. B., Schalekamp-Timmermans, S., Visser, W. E., Hofman, A., et al. (2015). Reference ranges and determinants of total hCG levels during pregnancy: the Generation R Study. *European Journal of Epidemiology*, 30(9), 1057–1066. doi: 10.1007/s10654-015-0039-0.

McGovern Medical School at The University of Texas Health Science Center at Houston (UTHealth).

Tomkins, Z. (2020). Endocrine system. In Z. Tomkins (Ed.) *Applied anatomy and physiology – an interdisciplinary approach.* (1st ed.) (pp. 169–194). Chatswood, NSW: Elsevier.

CASE 20
Breastfeeding challenges

HISTORY

Jade, who is 38 years old, has just given birth to her first child: a healthy baby boy, Billy. Following birth, Billy was placed on Jade's chest and the expectation was that Billy would latch onto the breast and start suckling. He did not do so. Instead, he looked curiously at his mother and the world around him. Although Jade had attended prenatal classes and was taught about how to breastfeed, she was not prepared for the possibility that the process would not work immediately. A midwife assisted with the process to help the mother and the infant to promote successful breastfeeding, but the baby still did not suckle. The midwife suspected that the baby would need more time to learn how to latch on, but also that the mother's milk was not yet available.

A decision was made to start bottle feeding while Jade was instructed on how to hand-express colostrum. The midwife assured Jade that, regardless of how much she expressed, the colostrum would be given to the infant. Jade was upset as she felt strongly that Billy should be breastfed and insisted on trying. However, after another quarter of an hour the baby did not latch on and was becoming upset. Jade agreed to try bottle feeding. Under the guidance of the breastfeeding consultant, Jade was able to produce a small amount of colostrum, which was immediately given to Billy via a syringe. During the following 24 hours, Jade and Billy continued to engage in the breastfeeding process. However, Billy still did not suckle despite Jade being able to produce a greater volume of breast milk, which in the end was given to Billy via bottle. Despite continuous efforts over the next 6 weeks of teaching Billy to latch on, the infant did not do so. Jade decided to continue to express breast milk for as long as possible. It also became evident in that time that Jade could not produce an adequate amount to support Billy's needs and it was necessary to supplement breastfeeding with baby formula. Despite Jade's efforts to regularly express milk, by 4 months after Billy was born Jade could hardly express

30 mL of milk. By four and half months after Billy's birth, Jade had ceased expressing milk as the expressed volume ranged between 5 and 10 mL. Billy continued with formula milk.

QUESTIONS

1. What is the physiological importance of a baby latching onto the mother's breast with respect to breast milk production?

2. What is the physiological importance of colostrum?

3. Discuss why Jade's capacity to produce breast milk decreased over time even though she regularly expressed milk via a breast pump.

4. At 4 months after birth, Jade's capacity to express milk had fallen to 30 mL per expression. Discuss why making the decision to stop would not impact Billy as much as if the decision had been made immediately after birth.

ANSWERS: CASE 20
Breastfeeding challenges

1. There are two main physiological events involved; both are driven by the endocrine system and are based on positive-feedback mechanisms. This means that the more the stimulus occurs the greater is the production of the hormone. The first physiological event is that of the oxytocin reflex – a mechanism that describes the effect of a positive mother–baby relationship on the secretion of oxytocin. In this case, placing Billy on Jade's chest straight after birth enabled Jade to touch, feel and smell her newborn. These events lead the posterior pituitary gland to release oxytocin. The second physiological event occurs when the baby latches onto the mother's breast. The suckling action stimulates mechanoreceptors in the areola to send signals to the hypothalamus to produce oxytocin and facilitate its release from the posterior pituitary gland (Figure 20.1). This hormone induces the contraction of myoepithelial cells located in the breast alveoli. The resulting reaction induces milk flow from alveolar epithelial cells to alveolar ducts, where it gathers for feeding. Milk is produced by lactocytes – cells found in the alveolar glandular epithelium. The suckling action also induces increased production of prolactin. This hormone is produced by the anterior pituitary gland and its main role is to regulate the secretion of breast milk from glandular epithelial cells in the breast alveoli. Prolactin is also proposed to have a relaxing and sleep-inducing effect on the mother despite the disruption of frequent nightly feeds. In this case, as Billy did not latch on, the positive-feedback mechanisms were not maintained.

2. Colostrum is the first form of the breast milk produced during late pregnancy and within a few days after giving birth. Although colostrum is produced in low volume, it is highly concentrated in nutrients, such as carbohydrates and protein, maternal leukocytes and antibodies. It is low in fat. Maternal leukocytes and maternal antibodies are the first immune protection the newborn has in the outside world. It is also proposed to have a mild laxative effect, which promotes the baby's intestines to pass the first stool (meconium). Breast milk is the first mode of establishing an infant's microbiome.

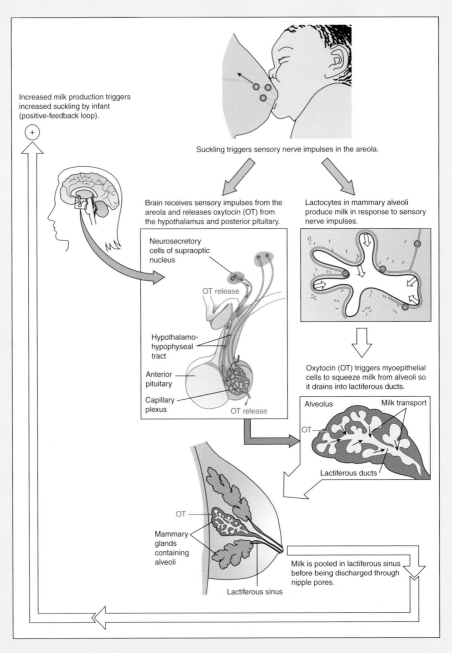

Increased milk production triggers increased suckling by infant (positive-feedback loop).

Suckling triggers sensory nerve impulses in the areola.

Brain receives sensory impulses from the areola and releases oxytocin (OT) from the hypothalamus and posterior pituitary.

Lactocytes in mammary alveoli produce milk in response to sensory nerve impulses.

Neurosecretory cells of supraoptic nucleus

OT release

Hypothalamo-hypophyseal tract

Anterior pituitary

Capillary plexus

OT release

Oxytocin (OT) triggers myoepithelial cells to squeeze milk from alveoli so it drains into lactiferous ducts.

Alveolus

Milk transport

OT

Lactiferous ducts

OT

Mammary glands containing alveoli

Milk is pooled in lactiferous sinus before being discharged through nipple pores.

Lactiferous sinus

FIGURE 20.1 A positive-feedback mechanism of infant breastfeeding on the release of oxytocin.

3. Although the literature is conflicting on whether the use of a breast pump can maintain breastfeeding as long as natural breastfeeding, the breastfeeding pump cannot replace the physiological effects of an infant suckling on the oxytocin reflex.

4. The most beneficial impact of the breast milk is in the early days as the infant adjusts to the new world. The colostrum and early milk provided the infant with immune protection and a highly caloric food source. When Jade decided to stop expressing milk owing to insufficient supply, the composition of the breast milk would not have provided the same protection as it did in first days of Billy's life. Had Jade made this decision at the time of birth, Billy would not have benefited from the beneficial effects of the colostrum.

BIBLIOGRAPHY

Bardanzellu, F., Fanos, V., Strigini, F., Artini, P. G., & Peroni, D. G. (2018). Human breast milk: exploring the linking ring among emerging components. *Frontiers in Pediatrics*, 6, 215. doi:10.3389/fped.2018.00215.

Carr, B. (2020). Pregnancy and lactation. In Z. Tomkins (Ed.) *Applied anatomy and physiology – an interdisciplinary approach.* (1st ed.) (pp. 399–414). Chatswood, NSW: Elsevier.

Feenstra, M. M., Jørgine Kirkeby, M., Thygesen, M., Danbjørg, D. B., & Kronborg, H. (2018). Early breastfeeding problems: a mixed method study of mothers' experiences. *Sexual and Reproductive Healthcare*, 16, 167–174. doi: 10.1016/j.srhc.2018.04.003.

Flagg, J., & Busch, D. W. (2019). Utilizing a risk factor approach to identify potential breastfeeding problems. *Global Pediatric Health*, 6, 2333794X19847923. doi: 10.1177/2333794X19847923.

Johns, H. M., Forster, D. A., Amir, L. H., & McLachlan, H. L. (2013). Prevalence and outcomes of breast milk expressing in women with healthy term infants: a systematic review. *BMC Pregnancy and Childbirth*, 13, 212. doi: 10.1186/1471-2393-13-212.

Marmet, C., Shell, E., & Aldana, S. (2000). Assessing infant suck dysfunction: case management. *Journal of Human Lactation*, 16(4), 332–336. doi: 10.1177/089033440001600409.

Tomkins, Z. (2020). Endocrine system. In Z. Tomkins (Ed.) *Applied anatomy and physiology – an interdisciplinary approach.* (1st ed.) (pp. 169–194). Chatswood, NSW: Elsevier.

INDEX

Page numbers followed by "*f*" indicate figures